PREGNANCY

— FOR —

DADS-TO-BE

Everything You Need to Know, from Conception to Birth

ADAM CARPENTER

Vie is an imprint of Summersdale Publishers Ltd

Summersdale Publishers Ltd
46 West Street
Chichester
West Sussex
PO19 1RP
UK

www.summersdale.com

Printed and bound in the Czech Republic

ISBN: 978-1-84953-819-0

Substantial discounts on bulk quantities of Summersdale books are available to corporations, professional associations and other organisations. For details contact Nicky Douglas by telephone: +44 (0) 1243 756902, fax: +44 (0) 1243 786300 or email: nicky@summersdale.com.

Disclaimer
Every effort has been made to ensure that the information in this book is accurate and current at the time of publication. The author and the publisher cannot accept responsibility for any misuse or misunderstanding of any information contained herein, or any loss, damage or injury, be it health, financial or otherwise, suffered by any individual or group acting upon or relying on information contained herein. None of the opinions or suggestions in this book is intended to replace medical opinion. If you have concerns about your partner's or your baby's health, please seek professional advice.

CONTENTS

INTRODUCTION

There is, I suspect, one common emotion that every man across the world feels to some degree when their other half utters those life-changing words: 'I'm pregnant.' Happiness? Joy? A teary-eyed appreciation of the miracle of life? Most likely that first emotion is pure, spine-tingling, stomach-churning, limb-shaking fear.

Well, dad-to-be, it's time to embrace this fear – and this book will help you to do it. First ask yourself just what it is that's making you feel this fear. Is it fear of the unknown? You know that in a few months' time your partner is having a baby but not very much about what goes on in between. The following chapters will guide you through the whole process, trimester by trimester.

Maybe it is money worries that are scaring you. If this is the case, then this book will advise what to buy, cutting out any unnecessary expenditure.

Or maybe it's the fear of losing your freedom? Hopefully this book will help you to realise over time that the joy of fatherhood is worth the change of lifestyle. Nothing else in your world will really compare to creating and nurturing a new life.

Another fear is of something going wrong. Of course it can happen, but out of the 700,000 babies delivered in England and Wales in 2013, just 5.9 per cent were miscarriages (unsurviving babies delivered before 24 weeks), with the figure for stillbirth (after 24 weeks) being under 0.5 per cent. We will discuss this topic but for the most part, this book presupposes that you will have a beautiful baby at the end of the pregnancy.

That's not to say it won't be a bumpy ride; over the next nine months or so, there will be tensions, worries and much uncertainty, but there will also be unforgettable memories to cherish, such as the moment you hear your baby's heartbeat for the first time.

And slowly you will feel more justified in saying: 'I am going to be a brilliant dad.'

So come on, don't be afraid. Let's do this!

CHAPTER 1
PREPARE YOUR PARTNER (AND YOURSELF) FOR PREGNANCY

Whether you are reading this book as a confirmed dad-to-be or a hopeful one, this first chapter will help you and your partner to prepare for a baby, however imminent this may be.

There are certain changes to your everyday routines that you can make that will not only help your partner cope more easily with the pregnancy and the birth but will also benefit the baby. You may have already made a start in this direction but, if not, it really isn't too late.

These changes apply equally if you are still trying to conceive and, of course, will be of continued benefit once your partner does fall pregnant.

Just as it is not too late to implement such changes, it is never too early to start preparing your home to accommodate a little person. This chapter will guide you through some of these preparations with the aim of helping you have less to do as the pregnancy progresses and avoid a last minute panic.

Of course, it's not all going to be so easy, and we will look at some of the obstacles you might face and how you can overcome them.

LIFESTYLE CHANGES

The lifestyle choices you make now won't just ensure a better start for your baby but they will also have long-term benefits for your and your partner's own health. Below are the lifestyle choices which require extra consideration during your partner's pregnancy.

SMOKING

Your partner has probably done so already, but have you stopped smoking? Or have you assured yourself that you won't smoke around your partner or the baby? Even second-hand smoke can reduce a baby's birthweight and it has been proven that it carries an increased risk of cot death, whilst more than 17,000 children under five are admitted to hospital every year due to the effects of second-hand smoke. Check out the Directory for an advice line number to help you or your partner to quit smoking.

ALCOHOL

Your partner is likely to have already stopped drinking by now – after all, what she drinks will make its way into your baby's bloodstream. According to NHS guidelines, drinking over one or two units a week while pregnant increases the risk of miscarriage, stillbirth and your baby being more prone to illness not just in childhood but throughout her life. If your partner is partial to a drink, seek out alternatives such as alcohol-free lager, ginger beer or an elderflower soda. Be considerate – stop drinking alcohol at home, curb your own social drinking (limit after-work drinks to once a fortnight) and find alternative ways of socialising with friends such as cinema trips. Your partner will really appreciate it.

CAFFEINE

Perhaps the one on the list that is easiest for us to forget, especially when doing the tea round! A moderate caffeine intake doesn't have any negative effects on your baby – it won't increase the chance of a miscarriage or cause any birth defects – but it will make it harder for your partner to absorb iron and calcium, both of which are good for the baby.

EXERCISE

If your partner is yet to fall pregnant, there are ways she can exercise to best prepare for the physical onslaught of carrying and delivering a baby – and you can support her by doing these exercises with her. Although, as always, she should run them past her doctor first, just in case there is a history of any problems that could be aggravated by doing these sorts of exercises.

It's the stomach that takes the most pounding during pregnancy so working on strengthening her deep abdominal muscles and the muscles in her lower back together will reduce back problems as the pregnancy progresses and perhaps even help her cope better with the labour itself. It will also make it easier to get her body back in shape once the baby arrives.

Think of your body as a core and these deeper muscles wrapping themselves around the spine, giving it support and strength like a corset. It's worth spending time to look up and master the exercises that will benefit these areas, or even consider enrolling in a yoga or Pilates class.

Toning the pelvic muscles will also help – they're the muscles we use to stop ourselves urinating, and by doing daily Kegel exercises, where you tighten these muscles and hold the contraction for three seconds, then release for three seconds, and repeat a few times, your partner is less likely to experience incontinence problems after she delivers.

Once your partner is pregnant, however, it is not advisable to start doing any strenuous exercise that she isn't used to doing. If, for instance, she wants to start an aerobics programme, make sure she starts slowly and informs her instructor that she is pregnant.

But exercise doesn't have to leave you exhausted to be beneficial – a simple half-hour's walk every day or swimming twice a week will contribute to a healthy lifestyle before, during and after pregnancy.

DIET

Preparing to become a parent is probably the best reason for both of you to eat healthily and, like all the above, it will benefit you all in the long term. If your partner is having issues with her weight – whether underweight or overweight – then encourage her to go to her GP for advice. But whatever your shape, everyone can benefit from a healthy eating plan.

Try eating a variety of fruit and vegetables every day. Processed foods often contain hidden salts and sugars, even if they purport to be good for you, and quite frankly, there is no need for them. Grilling a piece of meat or fish with some herbs for flavouring and steaming a few vegetables – even those in a microwaveable bag – is just as convenient, and possibly even quicker, than heating up a ready-made meal in the oven.

Eating protein-rich foods such as chicken and eggs will ensure normal growth of the baby and prevent a low birthweight. Protein will also keep your partner's body tissue in good shape.

In fact all the reasons for consuming food that is good for you apply in greater measure to your partner once she is carrying a baby. Keep up a good fibre intake as this will, among other benefits, reduce the risk for your partner of developing gestational diabetes.

Weight can be kept down by implementing small changes. Keep takeaways and desserts to a minimum. Even using olive oil instead of butter for frying and low-fat crème fraîche or yoghurt instead of cream in a recipe will help.

If you think none of this applies to you, keep a food diary for a week and you'll be surprised.

Healthy body = healthy sperm

If you and your partner are yet to conceive, there is a further incentive for you to stop smoking, curb your drinking and eat healthily. Sperm is just as affected by tobacco, alcohol, drugs and poor diet as are a woman's eggs. More fruit and vegetables in your diet improve the quality of your sperm because they contain antioxidants that prevent cell damage. Less junk food and fewer takeaways mean less excess weight, further helping your cause – one study of 2,111 couples experiencing fertility issues, conducted in 2006 by the US National Institute of Environmental Health Sciences, estimated a ten per cent increase in the likelihood of infertility for every 9 kg (20 lb) of excess weight.

Other factors that might affect sperm production are:

▶ **Regular use of hot tubs and saunas** – men are advised to keep their testicles at a temperature of around 34.5°C.

▶ **Excessive bike use** – putting pressure on the testes on a daily basis is again likely to keep the temperature inside higher than average.

▶ **Tight underwear** – this may hinder production, especially if sperm count is already an issue, so switch to loose-fitting boxer shorts.

THINGS TO BUY

There are some things that it's never too early to buy when you and your partner are planning to have a baby. If you haven't already done so, add the following to your shopping list:

FOLIC ACID SUPPLEMENTS

One tablet containing 400 mcg of folic acid a day is all your partner needs to significantly reduce your baby's risk of developing spina bifida – and the recommendation is that she starts taking it while trying to conceive, and keeps on taking it until she is full term. Once pregnant, she should get the supplements free on prescription.

Be wary about purchasing special 'pregnancy' multivitamins: according to NHS guidelines, the only other vitamin supplement needed during pregnancy – and not before it – is vitamin D. Other than that, a healthy balanced diet should provide you with all the essential vitamins and minerals. See the diet section on page 51, Chapter 2, for more information.

PREGNANCY TEST KITS

If you are still waiting for the magic blue line, it's worth investing in a supply of these. Shop online and you could buy a pack of 50, yes 50, pregnancy test strips for less than four quid – and that's for ultra-early test strips. At that price, your partner can check ten times over without breaking the bank. But, of course, before you go completely overboard, remember the ultimate pregnancy test is free on the NHS: your GP!

> **Top Tip**
>
> Pre-pregnancy, avoid the predictor kits which claim to tell your partner the best time to conceive. These can most definitely be filed under the box marked 'complete racket'. The best advice for conceiving – under normal circumstances – can be summed up in three words: just have sex!

A DECENT CAMERA

This is not the sort of purchase you are going to feel like splashing out on just as the baby is due and you still have a cot and pushchair to buy. Nor will you have much time on your hands to shop for one. So, if you don't already have one, treat yourself now and don't just save it to record baby's first entrance (actually don't record that – I meant to say baby's first *day*) but use it straight away for this precious time in your life as a couple when it is still just the two of you.

A HOUSE

If everyone waited until they were financially secure before having a baby, very few babies would be born. But if you are in a bedsit or a one-bedroom flat that is simply going to be too small once the baby comes along, do something about it now. If you're fortunate enough to be in a position to buy a property, find one that you can grow into. If you are renting, look for somewhere that will be right for you and the baby. Looking to move to a larger place when you have to – i.e. once there is a baby on the way – is not the most stress-free of options and there is no guarantee that you'll actually be in the larger place once the baby arrives.

PRE-PREGNANCY NESTING

The idea of nesting is something usually associated with women after they fall pregnant, which manifests itself in an obsession to organise the home in readiness for the new addition. But why not start now? The earlier you can plan your home around the possibility of starting a family by doing the following, the better...

GIVE YOUR HOME A THOROUGH CLEAN

The main aspect of nesting that your partner will develop once pregnant is a desire to clean. It is a primal instinct to have a safe environment for the new addition and that includes one that is clean. Plus it's a good mental boost to be surrounded by a clean and tidy space, especially if your partner has to spend more time in it later on in the pregnancy.

Now this isn't the 1950s and there is no excuse at all to simply let her get on with it while making jokes to your colleagues that it 'saves getting a cleaner in'. No, it's the twenty-first century and you're going to be the perfect partner and do your best to help.

Of course, you will already be sharing cleaning duties around the house (and if not, that's another thing you need to sort out), but I am talking about having a big top-to-bottom clean of your home – scrubbing cupboards inside and out, as well as surfaces, dusting all nooks and crannies. If you can afford it then employ the services of a cleaning company, but if not, it's time to get stuck in TOGETHER. Try to think of ways to make cleaning around the house easier such as decluttering areas or even investing in a more efficient vacuum cleaner – there won't be too much time to do it once the baby arrives but it will need to be done, especially in the first few weeks while your baby has to build up her immune system. The more you can tackle on this front before the baby comes, the better (and cleaner) life will be when you become parents.

HAVE A CLEAR-OUT

The moment your partner falls pregnant, your home will slowly fill up with baby paraphernalia and you will need to make room for it and for the baby when it arrives. So take a few trips to the tip and/ or charity shop with the stuff you know you no longer need or use. You'll feel better for it.

GET ORGANISED

You don't have to go quite as far as putting all the jars on the spice rack in alphabetical order but to give everything around the home its place – whether it's the paperwork, frying pans, toilet rolls – will, again, put you at a great advantage for the months ahead. Chances are one of you will be better at this sort of task than the other but it is probably worthwhile doing a certain amount together so you will both end up knowing where everything lives.

MIX MORE WITH FRIENDS WHO ARE PARENTS

Part of the process of nesting involves, a little brutally, having an almost unconscious sort-out of your friends. You will naturally see less of the ones without children and your partner in particular will most probably start making more contact with those who do have kids. Start this latter process as early as possible. You probably won't have seen as much of them since they became parents but they will appreciate the effort, even if it is just a quick meet-up for coffee or a simple phone call. Again, one day you'll appreciate a similar effort being made to come and visit you when you are surrounded by nappies and baby food all the time.

Doing this will help you acclimatise to the stage of your life that's ahead and get you in the mindset of what it is like to be around babies and toddlers. You don't have to go the whole hog and offer to babysit – although that will, of course, elevate your friends' appreciation for you to almost godlike status. And, who knows, they may return the favour someday.

UNDERSTAND HER FEELINGS

Helping with the practical stuff is just part of the story of being a dad-to-be. Doing your best to try to sympathise with how she is feeling and what her body and mind are going through at every stage is the real battle.

Never for one moment underestimate the changes your partner is facing as she embarks on carrying your baby. Here are some of the physical changes that she may be experiencing:

► Hair – the good news is that this gets thicker as pregnancy hormones stop it from falling out. There are, however, limits on the hair dye products and treatments that she can use. This may sound trivial to a bloke but to spend nine months with your roots showing can seriously undermine a woman's confidence and self-esteem.

▶ **Face** – along with the more obvious areas, such as stomach, legs and ankles, the face may swell and get rounder too due to fluid retention and the growing uterus putting pressure on the veins, slowing the return of blood to the heart.

▶ **Skin** – spots might appear and there could be possible changes in pigmentation, broken veins, chafing or, at the very least, itchiness. And don't forget the small matter of stretch marks as the baby grows and the stomach expands.

▶ **Breasts** – they get bigger and tender too, especially the nipples. Then at around 20 weeks into the pregnancy they gear themselves for milk production.

▶ **Bottom and thighs** – these will retain extra fat stores after the birth by way of preparing the body for breastfeeding.

▶ **Nails** – they'll grow more quickly but they will be more brittle than usual, so more manicures will be required.

This is all in addition to the astonishing thought that she is going to be carrying a little growing human inside her. So never lose sight, or understanding, of this immense scale of change that the woman you love is about to endure. And I didn't even mention the likelihood of morning sickness, heartburn, general discomfort and fatigue. Or the emotional stuff regarding the huge party inside her body that her hormones are about to have.

What are you doing still sitting here, man? Go and make her a cup of tea… then read on.

UNDERSTAND YOUR FEELINGS

Thus far a lot of this chapter has been all about your partner and not very much about you. It's worth remembering your feelings count too, and there will be moments when you will be entitled to be a little selfish – especially if you have been doing so much to make sure your partner is at her most comfortable and that consequently your baby is getting the best start.

It is important to take time out to do things that you want to do – but do make sure that you are upfront about it. Communicating your feelings to your partner at every stage is key – this isn't a time for bottling anything up. If something is worrying you regarding the implications a baby will have on your relationship or if you have fears about becoming a father, sure, you can talk them over with a friend or go online to a support forum, but the best way to deal with any such problems is to talk them over with your partner. This gives her the opportunity to listen and offer advice and understanding, and simply having the conversation will bring you closer together rather than the problem remaining a secret and pulling you ever so slightly apart.

PRE-PREGNANCY SEX

The good news is that one way to increase the likelihood of your partner getting pregnant is for you to have more sex. The bad news is sometimes you can have too much of a good thing – when the thought of conceiving becomes an obsession.

The reality is that in every month there is a relatively small window of opportunity for a sperm to fertilise an egg and it all centres around

Ovulation Day – the time when your partner's ovaries discharge their eggs, which then travel down the Fallopian tube where one may be met by a sperm and fertilised.

The big question is when this ovulation takes place. Well, it depends on two things…

1.   **The length of your partner's menstrual cycle**

2.   **How regular her periods are**

The menstrual cycle is the length of time between the first day of a woman's period to the day before her next. It is usually 28 days but can be as short as 22 and as long as 35. Ovulation usually happens around the halfway point of the cycle.

This is why it helps to know how regular your partner's periods are. If they vary from month to month it may be more difficult to pinpoint this important halfway point, but, approximately, you are talking about the end of the second week of the cycle and the start of the third being the most likely time that you are going to conceive.

So far, so unsexy. The general consensus is that the four to five days leading up to ovulation is when a sperm is most likely to meet an egg at ovulation – a woman's eggs normally survive for only 24 hours, whereas sperm can remain active for anything between three and five days. The most likely time for conception being the day before ovulation and the day itself.

Top Tip

If your partner is becoming anxious about conceiving, do make yourself available on the day before ovulation and the day itself – don't do what I did and be persuaded to go to the pub with the boss and only check your mobile to discover the increasingly irate 'Where are you?' texts at last orders! The fact is you are less likely to conceive if you are too anxious and obsessive about the whole thing.

Keep an eye on the important dates but just try to enjoy having sex. Make a night of it, create a romantic mood with dinner and massages, buy her sexy underwear, share fantasies and play around with positions and locations. If you're having fun, you will relax and be more likely to want to keep trying until you achieve the desired result.

WHEN THINGS DON'T GO ACCORDING TO PLAN

There are possible outcomes, both short-term and long-term, that need to be addressed.

WHAT IF WE CAN'T CONCEIVE?

When your hearts are set on being parents, it is hard when, after a few months, your partner still isn't pregnant. The simple thing is to say: 'Don't worry, it'll happen…' or 'It can take up to a year, you know…', but you'll soon get tired of hearing such words from people who know that you are trying.

In fact after about five months is the time at which it is a good idea to at least consider some of the possibilities that may be contributing to your fertility obstacles. So here is a summary:

Causes of infertility in both sexes

▶ **Sexually transmitted diseases such as chlamydia and gonorrhoea** – they're less likely, but still possible, in a long-term relationship but simple tests can rule them out.

▶ **Lifestyle issues** – such as smoking, alcohol and weight.

▶ **Chemicals and radiation in the workplace** – do you work in drug manufacture for cancer treatment, or work closely with X-rays or lead? These things don't always affect fertility but they carry risks.

Causes of male infertility

▶ **A lifelong illness** – such as thyroid disease or heart disease

▶ **Having mumps after puberty**

▶ **Erection problems**

▶ **Testicle issues** – have they been affected by tumours, cysts or cancer, or have you suffered a groin injury? Or maybe as a child, you had undescended testicles, where they don't move naturally into place in the scrotum after birth.

Causes of female infertility

Your partner will undoubtedly know these off by heart but let's run through them to get you up to speed.

- ▶ **Irregular or painful periods**

- ▶ **Polycystic ovary syndrome** – when the hormonal system gets out of balance, making ovulation rarer

- ▶ **Pelvic inflammatory disease** – an infection that can occur in the ovary, womb or Fallopian tubes, causing a blockage in the latter

- ▶ **Endometriosis** – when the endometrial cells lining the womb migrate to other parts of the body but act in the same way as those in the womb every month except the body struggles to discharge the resulting blood. A lot of cases (around 70 per cent) are quite mild and unproblematic but more severe instances can lead to a build-up of scarring, damaged ovaries or a blockage in the Fallopian tubes.

- ▶ **Fibroids** – non-cancerous tumours in the uterus, almost always benign but troublesome when it comes to conceiving

- ▶ **If she's had an ectopic pregnancy, where the embryo develops outside the womb** – if the embryo developed inside the Fallopian tube, it may have caused damage to the surrounding tubal tissue, meaning it is more likely that an egg will get stuck in the tube in future. It also depends on the condition of her other Fallopian tube.

- ▶ **Age** – fertility starts to decline in women from the age of 30, and after 35 it drops down more steeply. By 40, only two in five women wishing to have a baby will succeed.

In all these cases, if you suspect they might be contributing to your partner not getting pregnant, then see your GP.

Foods to help fertility

Aside from maintaining a healthy lifestyle, here are some of the superfoods that may help your partner to conceive:

▶ **Bananas** – these help regulate the hormones

▶ **Asparagus** – a good source of folic acid

▶ **Tofu** – good for iron, a lack of which may hinder ovulation

▶ **Salmon** – contains selenium which can prevent chromosome breakage

▶ **Peas** – good source of zinc to keep your hormones balanced

And a few for you to add to your diet:

▶ **Citrus fruit** – a natural boost of vitamin C will keep your sperm count high

▶ **Almonds** – contain vitamin E to improve sperm health

▶ **Mackerel** – the fatty acid DHA in fish oil also keeps your sperm healthy

▶ **Salmon** – that selenium may also make sperm more fertile

▶ **Peas** – zinc can boost sperm levels

MISCARRIAGE

Miscarriages are most common in the first 12 weeks of pregnancy, according to Tommy's, a charity that funds research into miscarriage, stillbirth and premature birth. Around 85 per cent of all miscarriages happen in this period. However, they must be mentioned in this first chapter as a great many of these occur before the woman has even realised she is pregnant.

But let's begin by saying that most pregnancies continue to full term, with miscarriage being more likely for those in the under 14 and over 40 age groups. So the odds are most definitely on your side for a straightforward pregnancy and a healthy baby.

Causes of miscarriage

Most early miscarriages are caused by the chromosomes of the foetus (another name for the very tiny developing baby). Chromosomes are blocks of DNA that contain detailed instructions of how the foetus will develop, from the colour of its eyes, how its cells will grow, etc. Sometimes something can go wrong at the point of conception and there is either too many or too few of these chromosomes. This prevents the foetus developing properly, leading to a miscarriage.

In other words, you often cannot predict or prevent this cruel process of nature, nor is it a sign that there is something wrong with the mother's or father's chromosomes. It is also comforting to know that such chromosome abnormalities are unlikely to recur when trying for another baby.

That said, the following will increase the risk of miscarriage:

▶ Smoking during pregnancy

▶ Drug misuse during pregnancy

▶ Drinking more than 200 mg of caffeine per day

▶ Drinking more than two units of alcohol a week

▶ Obesity

▶ Being underweight

Detecting a miscarriage

The first sign of a miscarriage is usually stomach pains and some bleeding – yet neither symptom is a definite indication of something serious. If bleeding happens in the first two or three weeks, it is more likely to be from the natural process of the fertilised egg burrowing into the lining of the uterus. Bleeding and cramping of the stomach is actually quite common throughout the first trimester, so it is important not to panic when this happens. If you are worried then call the midwife straight away as they will arrange an immediate appointment at the hospital to check that it isn't a miscarriage or, indeed, a sign of an ectopic pregnancy or an infection.

In the meantime, check for these other symptoms and phone the midwife IMMEDIATELY if your partner experiences any of the following:

▶ **Vaginal discharge like white-pink mucus**

▶ **Very painful cramps or contractions**

▶ **Sudden back pain**

▶ **Brown or bright red bleeding**

▶ **A clot-like discharge**

▶ **A drop in other pregnancy symptoms** – see more on pp.36–42 in Chapter 2

In addition to this, bleeding combined with the following symptoms may be a sign of an ectopic pregnancy. Again call the midwife immediately if your partner experiences any of the following:

- ▶ Severe pain in one side of the stomach

- ▶ Pain in the tip of a shoulder

- ▶ Diarrhoea or bowel pain

Equip yourself with these facts so you can ask the right questions in the event of your partner developing any symptoms that concern her – then phone the midwife who will arrange an appointment.

If for some reason you can't speak to the midwife over the phone, go straight to the accident and emergency department at your local hospital.

If your partner is bleeding, she should stem the flow with a tissue or put on a sanitary towel – under no circumstances should she use a tampon.

After miscarriage

In hospital, a scan will confirm the miscarriage – though in some cases, it may entail a few scans over a few days to be certain. A scan will also show up whether your partner will need a small operation known as an ERPC, which stands for the evacuation of retained products of conception.

Yet it is the emotional aftermath that will, understandably, take its toll and you may even find it hard to talk to each other about what has happened. Fortunately, there is help and support out there – for both of you – and a few numbers are given in the Directory at the back of this book.

Keep the lines of communication open between each other rather than bottling up your feelings, whether you are struggling to deal with feelings of grief, anger, guilt, envy of other couples who have babies or a mixture of some or all of these. And consider reaching out to a close friend or relative – or talk to your GP, who will be able to refer you to a bereavement counsellor. Research has shown that going down this path can significantly help you deal with your loss, so don't dismiss it.

And sooner or later you will want to decide on the right time to try again. Here you will have to take your partner's lead. Some women will want to try for a baby as soon as possible and in fact it may just happen. This doesn't mean they are not grieving for the one you have just both lost.

Others will be more explicit in their grief and need more time. The daily reminder of seeing other women who are happily pregnant or new mums pushing prams can be particularly hard to cope with, long after the physical loss is over. So you may need to give her time. Having sex may in itself also be an issue – regaining trust in her body, fears that she may suffer another miscarriage; these are all things that will hinder the process of moving on but, again, the key is to keep talking about your feelings to one another.

But hopefully soon – if she hasn't done so already – your partner will be telling you the good news that she is pregnant. To end this chapter on a positive note, there is one more important subject to cover…

TELLING PEOPLE YOU'RE EXPECTING

Of course, the news that your other half is pregnant is something that you are going to want to share with others, but don't go updating your Facebook status or pressing that 'send to all' button on your mobile just yet.

The accepted time for the Big Reveal is around the 12-week mark, after the first scan. By then, the risk of miscarriage has fallen dramatically and your other half's bump may begin to show.

Talk about the matter with your partner. It may be that she has already tweeted the news to her 687 followers! Equally she may be feeling anxious or simply superstitious about something going wrong if you tell people too early. Respect her wishes.

Here is a shortlist of people to share the news with at this early stage:

▶ **Close family** – you'll most probably want to tell your parents and siblings but make them aware if you are only telling a few people. You may feel that it goes without saying but say it anyway! It just takes the jungle drums of one overexcited relative and the news will be global before you know it.

▶ **Your boss** – it is best to inform your immediate line manager or supervisor that your partner is pregnant in the event of any unexpected hospital appointments, plus getting the time off for the 12-week scan can literally be done with a wink and a nod. Bosses are usually discreet – but if you can, choose the one you are most comfortable telling.

▶ **An understanding, (fairly) sensitive friend** – it wouldn't be fair for your other half to expect you not to tell anyone else! She will doubtless have someone close she'll be confiding in, so you should be fine picking one of your best mates too, whom you can share any worries with. It could be a pal who already has kids or is in a relationship where children are likely to be imminent – or, hey, it could be the 40-something barfly who still hasn't settled down but whose take on life will doubtless offer you some sense of clarity and perspective about the situation. There's merit in both!

As for anyone else – well, let them have fun guessing until you both decide to make a more general announcement. People love to say: 'I knew it!' when they finally find out.

In the meantime you've got plenty of other things to think about…

CHAPTER 2
THE FIRST TRIMESTER: 0–12 WEEKS

Having been given the news that you are going to be a dad, your head may very well be spinning with a variety of emotions, but time is on your side. There are months before your baby arrives and really begins to turn your life upside down. For you at least, the next few months are the easy bit. For your partner, it is always worth remembering, they are among the hardest. Chances are you will have found out about your forthcoming new addition at some point during the first 12 weeks of the pregnancy, or the first trimester. The word 'trimester' is actually a general word for 'a period of three months' that has over the years become synonymous with the three main stages of pregnancy.

Before we dive in and learn more of what each stage entails, it seems an ideal point to stop and take in just what is happening already in your unborn baby's world. Yes, they are still technically a foetus at 12 weeks but, wow, what a 12 weeks it has been.

The following should serve both to inform and maybe even impress a few of your mates when conversation dries up or, perish the thought, they actually start asking questions about your forthcoming fatherhood.

FACTS ABOUT YOUR BABY'S DEVELOPMENT

To get technical, the foetal development in humans actually begins around nine weeks. Before then your baby is still an embryo so the official term for development prior to this is embryogenesis. To confuse you further, for the first two weeks of pregnancy, your partner isn't actually pregnant – but the time is included in retrospect because it is the time from when she had her last menstrual period, a point which makes it helpful for the midwife to work out your baby's due date. It is during this fortnight that your sperm would have met your partner's egg as it was making its way from the ovary along the Fallopian tube to the uterus. Fertilisation happens in that tube and from there cells divide rapidly, forming the many cells that go to make a new individual. This means by the third week, a sonographer (the person who conducts ultrasound scans) can detect the start of life.

▶ Around **week three** the embryo starts growing a digestive tract, and the beginnings of what becomes an umbilical cord – which delivers nutrients and oxygen to the baby – can also be seen forming.

▶ By **week four**, the embryo has divided into three layers: the top one will soon sprout the brain, backbone and spinal cord; the middle one is starting to house the heart and circulatory system; the lower layer does the same for the lungs, intestines and the beginnings of the urinary system. And it's only the size of a poppy seed.

▶ Don't worry, though; at **week five** your embryo has its first growth spurt and balloons to a whopping – wait for it – 0.25 cm, resembling a tiny tadpole.

▶ At **week six**, your baby has an oversized head in proportion to the rest of its body and facial features are forming, including dark spots where the eyes will soon appear, openings where nostrils will be and pits from which ears will grow.

▶ The **week seven** mark will see the appearance of slightly webbed fingers and toes; 'This Little Piggy' renditions are still some way off.

▶ At **week eight** taste buds form on your baby's tongue, coinciding with the brain forming primitive neural pathways, thus small jerky movements on a sonogram are perfectly natural.

▶ **Week nine** and the embryonic tail has disappeared so your baby looks more human-like – wrists have developed, ankles have formed, arms have grown enough for elbows to form, whilst fingers and toes can be seen clearly. So sound the trumpets: a major milestone has been reached and your baby is no longer an embryo but a foetus – another word for 'offspring'. Genitals are even forming but it's too early to tell the sex.

From here your baby's development continues in force – their basic physiology being in place means they are poised for rapid weight gain.

▶ Just 3.1 cm long at **week ten** and yet your baby has a fully formed, though very dinky, set of organs – liver, kidneys, brain, intestines and lungs! A very detailed scan would even show up fingernails and hair.

▶ By **week 11**, all body parts from tooth buds to toenails are present and correct. Lots of kicking and stretching is taking place but it's too early for mum to feel anything.

► Now it's **week 12** and at 5.4 cm long, your baby's organs are hard at work: the liver is producing bile and the kidneys are secreting urine into the also-formed bladder. The baby's reflexes are good too – if you prod your partner's belly, the little one will most probably squirm.

WHAT HAPPENS TO YOUR PARTNER'S BODY?

Given all that your baby has achieved in the first 12 weeks, it should come as no surprise that your partner's body is having to work very hard. Here is a rundown of what's happening to her:

► **Early pregnancy** signs include tender breasts, tiredness and nausea – all of which could simply indicate another period is coming up.

► **By four weeks**, the need to wee will become more frequent and there may be cramps and bleeding from the embryo implanting itself in the womb.

► **Between five and eight weeks** is when morning sickness could arise, coupled with a change in the tastes and smells that your partner likes. Heartburn and erratic mood swings could also be prevalent.

► Thus far a pregnancy hasn't really shown but **from nine to 12 weeks**, the waistline starts to expand. Some women experience constipation which can be reduced by drinking plenty of water and adopting a high-fibre diet. Craving certain foods isn't uncommon.

DEALING WITH FIRST TRIMESTER HEALTH CONDITIONS

Throughout pregnancy there are a variety of symptoms that your partner will develop, some specific to certain trimesters, whilst others may occur in all three with varying degrees of severity.

Here are the ones that she is most likely to encounter in the first trimester and how you can help her deal with them:

BLEEDING

What causes it? Arguably the most concerning symptom of early pregnancy will, in the majority of cases, cause no harm to the baby whatsoever. It happens to around 1 in 5 women, usually at the time that their period would be due, and may last for a couple of days. Here are possible reasons for bleeding:

▸ Pregnancy hormones may be covering up the usual menstrual cycle, leading to what is known as breakthrough bleeding.

▸ It could simply be a result of the fertilised egg implanting itself in the uterus. This is known as implantation bleeding.

▸ The cervix is softening, causing a raw area to form that may be vulnerable to bleeding.

▸ A vaginal or cervical infection.

▸ A harmless growth such as a polyp.

▸ Chafing of the cervix, possibly after sex.

What should I do? Don't panic but do contact your GP or midwife, who may refer your partner to an Early Pregnancy Assessment Unit (EPAU). They also might refer to this as a 'threatened miscarriage' but again this is not a reason to get even more concerned, just an indication that they are taking the matter seriously.

At the EPAU, your partner will have her blood and urine tested to check pregnancy hormone levels and her cervix will be examined to check that it is closed.

She may also be given an ultrasound scan to check the baby's heartbeat. In most cases, everything will be OK but if there is a problem, you will be in the right place to receive treatment at the earliest opportunity.

When will it stop? Bleeding in early pregnancy may recur later in pregnancy but many mums-to-be who experience it go on to have healthy babies.

MORNING SICKNESS

What causes it? Around seven out of ten women will be affected by this in the early stages of pregnancy. Morning sickness can actually occur at any time of the day (or night) and as early on as three weeks after conception – in some cases, it is what alerts a woman to the possibility that she could be pregnant.

The nausea could be a result of her rising levels of oestrogen and progesterone, which cause the stomach to empty more slowly. Also she has a heightened sense of smell so strong food odours, tobacco smoke or deodorants might all make her feel nauseous.

What should I do? Most cases of nausea can be eased by adhering to the following:

▶ Put the pungent curries on hold for a while and pick foods low in fat and easy to digest, such as chicken.

▶ Having smaller meals more often throughout the day will also stop her feeling so full, so think of snacks that might fit this ideal such as hummus and vegetables. Eating regularly like this will also stave off hunger, which is another thing that can make the nausea worse.

▶ Remember the particular foods that set off her nausea and avoid buying them!

▶ Plenty of fluids will help ease the sickness. And have a ready supply of ginger ale as that helps too. Iced water and barley water are also good.

▶ In more extreme cases, you can try motion sickness bands, hypnosis, aromatherapy (peppermint is a good scent to ease nausea) and even acupuncture, but check with your GP or midwife first.

However, you should take your partner to see the doctor if the nausea is severe and she is experiencing any of the following:

▶ Struggling to keep fluids down

▶ Having dizzy spells

▶ Vomiting blood

▶ Not passing much water or if her urine is dark in colour

When will it stop? Around the fourteenth week of pregnancy is when most cases of morning sickness cease, although it isn't unusual for it to last a little longer.

So what was it that the Duchess of Cambridge suffered? That was hyperemesis gravidarum, which is the name for excessive nausea and vomiting. If your partner is being sick several times a day and unable to keep any food or drink down, she is likely to need hospital treatment. There is a severe risk of dehydration and weight loss with this condition so, before either of these can happen, contact your GP or midwife, or just take her straight to hospital. The treatment will set her right but bear in mind that this type of sickness can last up to the twentieth week and in some cases won't clear up completely until the baby is born.

HEARTBURN AND CONSTIPATION

What causes it? In order that your unborn baby receives the nutrients it needs from your partner, pregnancy actually slows down the movement of food through her digestive system so these nutrients have more time to be absorbed into the bloodstream and therefore reach the womb. Except this process also causes constipation. Meanwhile, it increases the chances of heartburn as the body also relaxes the valve between the stomach and oesophagus, which allows stomach acid to leak into the oesophagus.

What should I do? Again it comes down to diet. Heartburn can be prevented by having smaller meals more frequently throughout the day and avoiding foods that are higher in fat and anything spicy, plus no carbonated drinks or citrus fruits and juices. Constipation can be relieved by eating foods high in fibre, such as stewed prunes, and also by drinking lots of fluids. Exercising regularly will also help.

When will it stop? Heartburn potentially can carry on throughout the whole pregnancy but it is easily preventable. The same goes for constipation – if you think about it, the baby is going to need nutrients throughout its time in the womb.

DIZZINESS

What causes it? Pregnancy dilates the blood vessels and lowers blood pressure, both of which may cause light-headedness and dizziness.

What should I do? There are a few quite simple things for you to keep in mind to help beat the dizzy spells:

▶ Make sure your partner isn't standing for prolonged periods – hence why she and other pregnant women need that seat on the bus!

▶ If she feels dizzy, get her to lie down on her left side or sit with her head between her knees to improve blood flow to the brain. Also she should rise slowly after she has been sitting or lying down.

▶ Dizziness may also be a sign that she is hungry and her blood sugar level has dropped so prepare her an appropriate snack.

▶ If she has prolonged bouts of dizziness and it occurs with abdominal pain and vaginal bleeding, seek medical care. It could be an indication that she is having an ectopic pregnancy, where the fertilised egg implants itself on the outside of the uterus. This could be life-threatening if left untreated.

When will it stop? It should ease by the end of the first trimester as her body adjusts to the changes, but later in the pregnancy the uterus will grow large enough to put pressure on her blood vessels so dizziness could potentially be a regular occurrence until birth.

ANXIETY

What causes it? The emotional strain of being pregnant must never be ignored. Imagine if you were suddenly given the news that another human being was growing inside your body. That for the next eight or nine months, whatever you do will have some sort of impact on this tiny little thing. You'd be a little worried, to put it lightly.

Well, that is exactly what your partner is having to deal with – and it is such a huge responsibility. No matter how much support you both have around you, no matter all the reassurances you can give her, ultimately she is the one who is going through it all and whose day-to-day behaviour has a significant effect on how healthy your child turns out to be. No surprise, then, that you may find that your partner starts crying or experiencing mood swings for no apparent reason.

What should I do? You have to train yourself to respond in a sensitive and understanding manner and remember that she is pregnant and this most probably accounts for such behaviour. So no losing your temper or rolling your eyes or making any sarcastic or cutting remarks – even if you might be having a heated discussion or argument (though try keeping these to a minimum). Instead, encourage her to communicate. In other words, your reaction to any weeping episode or mood swing should be to ask 'What's wrong?' or 'How are you really feeling?' These are questions that don't just require a few words as an answer and for conversation to move on. They invite your partner to sit down with you, knowing that you will take the time to listen as she says what is worrying her at that moment. It could be anything – from financial worries about having a baby to the effect it may have on your relationship to how motherhood is going to impact her career.

When will it stop? This one will obviously run all the way through the pregnancy but the good news is that she will most definitely stop worrying about your unborn baby after giving birth. Instead it switches to worrying about your baby in the outside world – luckily, though, she'll have you to share the worry and responsibility that is unlikely to stop for the next 18 years. At the very least...

OTHER SYMPTOMS AND QUICK FIXES

Symptom: Tender breasts
Quick fix: A few new bras wouldn't go amiss – but get her to tell you the right size!

Symptom: Fatigue
Quick fix: Though it's obvious to see that she rests as much as she can, exercise such as a short brisk walk will help keep the tiredness at bay and stop it dominating her day-to-day life.

Symptom: Increased urination
Quick fix: If going out and about, check that a toilet won't be too far away. Your partner should also avoid any food and drink containing caffeine late at night.

Help prevent back pain

Now more than ever you must set your gentlemanly behaviour barometer to the max. If there are shopping bags to be carried or washing baskets to be lifted, you should be the person to do it. Of course, you can't be around your partner 24/7 and you don't want to fuss every time she so much as lifts a few magazines off the coffee table, but keep an eye out for ways that you can make sure she isn't exerting herself. Back pain can become a problem during pregnancy and the more you can do to alleviate this, the better.

ANTENATAL CARE

Wherever you happen to be registering on the 'nervous about becoming parents' scale, it is reassuring to know that there is a great deal of support available to your partner – and you – at every stage of the pregnancy through the NHS. For first-time pregnancies, there will be about ten antenatal appointments throughout the whole nine months – with that figure reducing to seven for women who have given birth before.

If your partner has – or develops – a medical condition, she will, of course, have more appointments. Rest assured she and your baby are well looked after from now on – and if, for whatever reason, you ever feel that this isn't the case, speak up to a member of NHS staff until someone listens.

Below is a summary of the two main appointments that crop up in the first trimester, to give you a rough idea of dates for your diaries.

THE FIRST VISIT

When? In the first few days of pregnancy, after your GP has confirmed that you are pregnant.

What for? To officially register your partner as pregnant and check her general health.

What will it tell us? Your partner will be given information about the importance of a healthy diet, taking folic acid supplements and giving up smoking, drinking and drugs. Yet it's a worthwhile checklist to go over at any stage and if you or your partner are having difficulty with any of these issues, extra help is available. The visit will also enable your partner to mention any medical conditions that might have an impact on the pregnancy and require further support. These include:

- ▶ Diabetes
- ▶ A history of high blood pressure
- ▶ If a family member has a baby with an abnormality, such as spina bifida
- ▶ If there is a family history of an inherited disease, such as cystic fibrosis
- ▶ Complications or infections that arose in a previous pregnancy such as pre-eclampsia or a premature birth

This list is by no means exhaustive, so your partner should mention any medical condition that she feels might affect the pregnancy in some way, even if it is to seek reassurance that it will not.

Should I be there? No – in fact your partner will probably be advised to attend this alone as some women feel more comfortable discussing sensitive matters, such as any of the above medical conditions, without having their partner in attendance. It makes it easier for the GP or midwife to ask the appropriate questions too.

THE BOOKING APPOINTMENT

When? Around eight to 12 weeks.

What for? This is the first official appointment and usually takes place at a health centre or in a hospital and will be with a midwife or doctor.

What will it tell us? The midwife or doctor will want to build up a picture of how the pregnancy is progressing thus far so they can identify any risks at the earliest opportunity and deal with them accordingly. There will be another recap on the importance of a healthy diet and lifestyle but you will also be given further information on pelvic floor exercises and other ways for your partner to keep her body in as good a shape as possible throughout pregnancy.

You will be told more about just how your baby is developing and the services that the NHS provides, including antenatal screening tests, antenatal classes and breastfeeding workshops. It is also a good opportunity to pick up more information about benefit entitlement and even planning the actual labour. It's never too early to think of this, so take a look at the options available to allow time for plenty of discussion on the matter.

It is a lot to take in for one appointment and doubtless there will be questions that you will both want to ask – writing them down beforehand will be a big help.

Should I be there? Yes. This will be an opportunity, in some cases, for you to have a blood test to ascertain whether there are any inherited conditions on your side that you may not know about and that might affect the baby. Also, with a lot of ground to cover, the appointment can take up to two hours and, if nothing else, it would be nice for your partner to have the company and a hand to hold.

But, above all, this could be (though not necessarily) the first moment that you will be seeing an image of your baby flashing up on screen. A tiny dot flickering on a murky image may not sound like much of a reason to miss a morning at work but, trust me, it is an incredible, unforgettable experience.

THE DATING SCAN

When? Usually around 12 weeks, after you have had the booking appointment.

What's it for? Your partner has an ultrasound scan so the midwife can give you the date when the baby will be at full term.

What will it tell us? The most likely date when your lives will truly change forever, give or take a few days either side. Oh, and the scan should also reveal if your partner is having twins (though if she was given a scan at the booking appointment, you may already know this).

Should I be there? Of course! Do you really just want to receive a still from the scan by email while you're at work? You'd have told your supervisor/boss in good time so make the effort to be there. The news should be good so it should be a day to remember and celebrate.

ANTENATAL CLASSES

Why? These are designed to help your partner – and you – prepare for the baby's birth and also learn to look after and feed the baby.

Woah, what already? Don't worry! The classes don't normally start until your partner is around the 30-week mark but it is worth signing up for them now to ensure you get registered on the one(s) that you want, because places can get snapped up early. Speak to your GP or midwife about them or contact the charity NCT (formerly the National Childbirth Trust), although NCT classes are somewhat expensive considering the NHS equivalents are free.

Should I be there? Yes! There's a lot of information that will prove handy when labour day arrives – from practical things such as where you can park at the hospital to breathing exercises that you can help her with in between the contractions. It's also an opportunity to meet other dads and mums in your area who are going to have this amazing life-changing experience around the same time as you. The potential for lifelong bonds for you, your partner and child might just begin here. So make sure your partner books them for a time that fits around your work.

THE 'EATING FOR TWO' MYTH

Now that you know the baby is on its way for sure, you and your partner will be keen to add those foods to the shopping list that are known to have health benefits for your partner and your baby.

The important thing to remember is that the age-old adage that she is 'eating for two' now is simply not true. Imagine a baby sitting at the dinner table with you – would you seriously serve up the same portions as you would to an adult?

Here are a few facts to further dispel the myth:

▶ Your partner needs about 300 extra calories a day.

▶ 300 calories is the equivalent of a slice of wholegrain bread and a tablespoon of peanut butter.

▶ Based on the recommended 2,000 calories per day for a woman, she is, at most, 'eating for one and a seventh'.

▶ Overeating during pregnancy not only increases the risk of gestational diabetes later on in pregnancy, as well as backaches and high blood pressure, but if the baby puts on too much weight, your partner is more likely to need a Caesarean.

So how much weight should your partner be putting on throughout the pregnancy? The official measurement of weight is the body mass index (BMI) which correlates your height and weight to give an estimate of proportion of body fat.

▶ If your partner's BMI was between 18.5 and 24.9 pre-pregnancy, she is at a healthy weight and should gain anything between 11 kg and 16 kg (25 lb and 35 lb) throughout the whole pregnancy.

▶ If your partner's BMI was between 25 and 29, she is classed as overweight and she should be looking to gain between 7 kg and 11 kg (15 lb and 25 lb) throughout the whole pregnancy.

▶ If your partner's BMI was 30 or over, she is classed as obese and should be looking to gain anything between 5 kg and 9 kg (11 lb and 20 lb) throughout the whole pregnancy.

▶ Oh, and not forgetting twins. If you're expecting twins, these figures increase to between 17 kg and 25 kg (37 lb and 54 lb) if your partner started at a healthy weight, between 14 kg and 23 kg (31 lb and 50 lb) if she was overweight, and between 11 kg and 19 kg (25 lb and 42 lb) if she was obese.

If your partner falls in the overweight or obese category, she is not alone – around half of all pregnant women do. Needless to say, there is plenty of help out there to ensure that they consume the number of calories that they need and don't go over (or under) that level. Don't let the burden fall on your partner's shoulders – adjusting your eating habits and introducing an exercise routine is something you can, and must, work on together. Speak to your GP, midwife or other health professional and they will point you in the right direction.

It's a sensitive issue and you may have to tread carefully. A lot of women at some point in their lives suffer from hang-ups and anxiety about eating and how it affects their weight and pregnant women are no different. Just because she has found out she is carrying a baby doesn't suddenly banish a woman of the worry that her bum is big or stop her from feeling like she has a spare tyre for a belly. If anything it may make it worse.

Be extremely gentle in raising the subject of possibly seeking some help if you think it applies and reassure her that it isn't just about doing it for the baby but also about helping her change her life in the long term. Remember, pregnancy is not the time to go on a weight loss diet. For your partner to restrict calories is potentially dangerous to her and the baby, so do seek medical help.

Top Tip

It is worth emphasising just how much of a myth the 'eating for two' saying is. If I had my time again, I would certainly have helped my wife to eat more healthily throughout both her pregnancies. I'm not saying I gave her two chocolate bars instead of one every time we stopped for coffee but I just wish we had paid more attention to the quality and quantity of foods we were eating – for instance, it was around the time the supermarkets had started selling those takeaway curries in a bag and it is only in retrospect we have realised how immensely calorific they are, when actually it isn't too much effort to make a home-made curry that is much healthier and tastier too. Also, you are more likely to make smaller portions at home compared to these ready-made bags that say they serve two but have enough for three. I think subliminally you can easily slip into the 'eating for two' mentality and assume the weight will drop off later but that is just not the case.

Once the baby comes along and requires 24/7 care, your partner will have very little time to devote to exercising, let alone the energy or inclination in those rare free hours she has.

We're not talking about dieting. Choosing a grilled sardine salad instead of a plate of fish and chips is not dieting. You reach for a banana instead of a doughnut because you are set upon eating healthily, not because you are looking to lose weight.

THE DANGERS OF DIETING IN PREGNANCY

Dieting – i.e. consuming less than the recommended number of calories – during pregnancy is as much fraught with dangers as is overeating. It can lead to a low birthweight and premature delivery, both of which can go on to cause developmental delays, learning disabilities and chronic health problems in your baby. In extreme cases, it can prove fatal to the baby.

So get dieting out of your partner's head completely. Even if her BMI is 25 or above, the good news is that there is still no need for her to go on a diet. In the first trimester it is common to actually lose weight due to morning sickness. Obviously this is an unpleasant thing to go through but on the plus side being sick reduces the intake of calories and the nausea will likely diminish her appetite.

And adopting a pregnancy-friendly, health-professional-approved diet at this stage will mean you can stop gaining too much weight whilst still having enough of a store of body fat in reserve to give your baby everything a growing foetus needs.

FOODS TO EAT AND FOODS TO AVOID

Below is a list of some of the foods that contain nutrients that will benefit your partner and the baby, particularly in the first trimester. Add them to the shopping list if you haven't already done so and remember you don't have to overdo them. Just eat them as part of that balanced healthy diet you have already adopted:

▶ **Eggs** – one a day will boost protein levels as well as vitamins A and B12 and choline, which recent research suggests may help foetal and infant brain development, influence memory and learning ability in later life and even protect against spina bifida. **But ensure the eggs are well cooked** (see p.53). Other sources of protein include: lean chicken or beef, nuts, cheese.

▶ **Berries** – including strawberries, blueberries, blackberries or cherries – act as antioxidants that rid the body of cell-damaging free radicals.

▶ **Plain yoghurt** – a great source of zinc and calcium, particularly good if your partner can't bear the thought of drinking milk.

▶ **Prunes** – a great source of fibre, which keeps your partner's digestive system in tip-top condition. Fibre can also reduce the chance of developing pre-eclampsia. Other sources of fibre: pulses, wholegrain and oranges.

▶ **Spinach** – a great source of folic acid/folate that will help protect against spina bifida. Other sources of folate include broccoli and sweet potato.

▶ **Salmon, haddock and cod** – lower in fat than most meat, these types of seafood contain high levels of omega-3 which will keep your partner's heart healthy and help your baby's brain to develop. Hate fish? Avocado contains omega-3 too.

▶ **Chia seeds** – these are worth seeking out and sprinkling over your cereal every morning as they contain good levels of fibre and omega-3 fats, but also they inhibit the speed at which sugar is absorbed into the body, meaning your baby can grow with fewer mood swings caused by spikes in blood sugar levels.

And the foods to strike off the shopping list for sure (at least as far as your partner is concerned):

▶ **Soft cheeses with white rind**, such as Brie and Camembert and certain goat's cheeses, have been mould-ripened and may contain harmful bacteria such as listeria which causes listeriosis and is highly dangerous for the baby.

▶ **Soft blue cheeses** such as Danish blue and Gorgonzola must also be avoided for the same reason.

▶ **All types of pâté**, including vegetable pâté, can contain listeria.

▶ **Raw and undercooked eggs** could contain salmonella, which won't usually harm the baby but will, of course, give your partner a severe bout of food poisoning. So hard boil those eggs and avoid home-made mayonnaise and cake and biscuit dough that contains raw eggs.

▶ **Raw and undercooked meats** carry a very small risk of toxoplasmosis that can harm the baby, but it is very hard to detect as there are no symptoms. So cook all meats until the juices run clear and wipe surfaces and wash hands thoroughly after handling raw meats. For a similar reason it is best to avoid cured meats such as salami and chorizo unless you are cooking them.

▶ **Liver** contains too much vitamin A which can harm your baby.

▶ **Shark, swordfish and marlin** are all bad on the seafood front as they contain mercury which will affect your baby's nervous system. For that reason, your partner shouldn't have more than two tuna steaks or four tins of tuna in any one week. Also two tuna steaks will put your partner at the ideal limit for oily fish (including fish oil supplements) so have no more of any variety in that week.

▶ **Raw shellfish** is prone to harmful bacteria that might cause food poisoning. Cooked thoroughly, however, they are fine.

The following are safe:

▶ **Cream cheese**

▶ **Halloumi, feta cheese, mozzarella**

▶ **Peanuts**

▶ **Milk and other dairy products** – as long as they have been pasteurised

▶ **Ice cream** – again the ingredients should have been pasteurised

▶ **Liquorice**

ALCOHOL IN PREGNANCY

In February 2015 the Royal College of Obstetricians and Gynaecologists (RCOG) updated their guidelines to say that abstinence is the only way to ensure that your baby is not harmed by alcohol. Previously it had stated that up to two glasses of wine a week was acceptable but now the group recognises that the time around conception and the first three months of pregnancy is when an unborn baby is most at risk from harm as a result of even a small amount of alcohol.

In extreme cases – where the mother has regularly been binge drinking throughout early pregnancy – alcohol can increase the chance of a miscarriage.

Continuing to drink alcohol can have a serious list of implications for your growing baby. Alcohol can pass via the placenta from the mother's blood into the baby's blood and can damage the growth of its cells. Brain and spinal cord cells are most likely to be affected.

Of course, it isn't worth worrying about how much alcohol your partner has consumed while she didn't know she was pregnant – the chances are extremely high that no damage would have been done. However, if she has been drinking heavily on a regular basis and she is struggling to curb her drinking or she has an ongoing alcohol addiction, talk to your GP. Your partner mustn't feel that your GP is going to be judgmental or disapproving. They will have dealt with a pregnant woman in the same situation numerous times before. So go and see them – go with your partner to the appointment, even if you don't actually go into the doctor's room with her, although it's probably more useful if you do because you can tackle the problem together. Really, you won't be the first to approach your GP with this problem and the sooner you tell them about any issues with alcohol, the sooner they can help you to do something about it.

Even if your partner has no issues relating to alcohol misuse, you can support her by giving up drinking around the house. No one is going to frown on you for going out to the pub with colleagues once in a while – and your partner will enjoy having a gloat when you wake up with a hangover the next morning. Less acceptable is you cracking open some Pinot Grigio in front of the television whilst she is sadly nursing her third glass of barley water of the night.

EXERCISE

IMPORTANT NOTE

Before taking up any new form of exercise, check with your midwife/
GP to make sure there are no harmful effects for the mother or baby.

The thought of doing any exercise while pregnant is probably an alien concept to some. Surely being pregnant takes it all out of a woman – the tiredness, the sickness, the physical discomfort. And how do you know that the exercise she's doing isn't going to harm her unborn baby? Yet carried out correctly and sensibly, certain exercise will help keep common pregnancy symptoms such as fatigue, backache and constipation at bay.

It will also help keep blood sugar levels steady if your partner develops gestational diabetes later on in pregnancy. Plus it's good for the mind, boosting her self-esteem and making her less prone to depression.

What's more, exercise will keep the weight gain down and prepare body and mind for labour and birth – potentially reducing the length of time that it takes to actually give birth.

In short anything you can do to help your partner exercise will potentially have long-term benefits throughout and beyond pregnancy, and crucially in the first few months after the baby is born when the absence of time in which to exercise will be compounded by the feeling that she is never going to shift the baby weight. If you've taken steps to conquer this early on, it's a real boost on the self-esteem front.

Don't overdo your encouragement in this to the point of nagging – think of yourself as more personal training pal than personal trainer and do what you can to make exercising fun and part of your week-to-week routine.

Below are the best exercises to do in the first trimester:

▶ **Brisk walking and swimming** are both good for helping your partner get a good night's sleep so long as you don't exercise too late in the day. An early evening walk or swim is perfect to make her feel comfortably tired by bedtime – and it is a pleasant activity that you can do together.

▶ **Pregnancy yoga and Pilates** are both good for strengthening and toning muscles, keeping the weight gain at bay, but find a qualified instructor who is experienced in teaching pregnant women.

▶ **Pelvic floor exercises** can help reduce the strain on the pelvis and relieve back pain. Just a few a day can really help prevent bladder weakness and prolapse symptoms.

▶ **Lifting weights** might not seem appropriate for your partner or the baby but light weights to keep the arms and legs toned will make her more able to move around in a few months' time when her bump will be approaching full size. Post-pregnancy, a toned body helps to make carrying round a growing baby/toddler far easier.

So how much exercise is good? A 30-minute session of manageable exercise three times a week is a good target – or three 10-minute sessions throughout a day instead – but if she can do a little more throughout the week, all the better. Light household chores or even having a bit of a bop in the lounge all contribute to the greater cause.

Here are a few important dos and don'ts that your partner should remember…

▶ DON'T overdo it – a good guideline is that your partner should still be able to talk comfortably while exercising.

▶ DO vary the exercise routine – a mix of aerobic exercise to work the heart and lungs and keep calories down, coupled with strength and conditioning exercises to work those muscles and regulate toning is ideal.

▶ DON'T embark on contact sports, such as ice hockey or basketball, where she may get hit in the stomach. Also avoid sports where there is a risk of falling such as horse riding and skiing, and high-altitude exercise such as mountaineering, where less oxygen means less oxygen for the baby, and also increases the likelihood of dizziness and tiredness. Of course, there are people who will argue otherwise, but doing without these sports for nine months to be on the safe side is not that big a deal.

▶ DO make sure she listens to her body – the first complaint of feeling too tired, faint or dizzy, then she should stop.

▶ DO encourage your partner to continue with any fitness classes or routines that she did pre-pregnancy, such as running or using the gym. It is important to keep up her fitness levels, so long as she doesn't overdo it. Plus there are ways to help adapt to a growing bump such as wearing appropriate exercise wear that will support and protect the bump. She can speak to her GP or midwife if she has any concerns.

▶ DON'T continue with high-energy workouts such as heavy weightlifting, long-distance running, etc. Such activities are likely to put stress on the joints and pelvic floor muscles.

▶ DON'T exercise in humid conditions. It is important her body doesn't overheat, especially in the first trimester when the body struggles to regulate its temperature. Make sure she's cool and drinking water as often as is sensible. And if she is swimming, make sure the pool isn't over 32°C. Most leisure pools are below this, although you may wish to check if you are abroad.

▶ DO encourage her to talk to her GP before undertaking any exercise if she has experienced any of the following: high blood pressure, joint or muscle problems, heart or lung problems, anaemia, premature birth or threatened miscarriage. She should also talk to her GP if her BMI is 12 or lower or 40 or higher.

▶ DON'T exercise if expecting twins or indeed more – consult the midwife for advice before exercising.

But now to an altogether different exercise – and it is worth remembering it is exercise…

SEX

After the fun part of trying to conceive, it can be difficult for a man to adjust to the idea of having sex with his partner now that she is pregnant. You might worry that you are going to harm the baby – or your partner – but in most cases sex at any stage of pregnancy is perfectly safe. The foetus is surrounded by the muscles in the uterine walls and by the abdomen. There is also a sac of amniotic fluid which further protects the baby. Plus if you are concerned that your penis is going to go in too far, there is a mucus plug making the cervix (the neck of the womb) completely impassable.

Of course, there are exceptions. Your partner should speak to her GP on the subject of whether it is advisable to have sex if:

- ▶ she has a history of miscarriage.

- ▶ she has had complications with previous pregnancies.

- ▶ she experiences vaginal bleeding.

- ▶ she develops stomach cramps.

Check YOUR sexual history

Can you be sure you are not carrying a sexually transmitted infection such as chlamydia or herpes? Depending on how long you have been with your partner, it may be that you could have caught something in a previous relationship that could cause problems with your current partner's pregnancy. Some research suggests chlamydia, for instance, can increase the risk of miscarriage, premature birth or stillbirth – so get yourself tested.

Provided that none of the above is stopping you, then here are some reasons why you and your partner SHOULD be having sex at this stage of pregnancy:

► **Heightened pleasure** – increased blood flow to the pelvic area can cause engorgement of the genitals. This can work in one of two ways – it could add to her pleasure during sex but equally it might leave her feeling uncomfortably full and in need of the toilet.

► **Strengthened emotional connection** – you're having a baby together! Wow! The emotional bond between you is growing, even if you haven't had much chance to think about it. Well, think about it as you make love, when you will most likely want to hold her, look at her, and kiss her, and just see how it makes you feel. Sex during pregnancy can do more than just keep your relationship alive – it can really enhance it.

► **Good for the baby** – if something makes mummy feel good, then chances are that she will pass on those feel-good hormones to the baby. Sex is a known stress buster and that alone is a positive thing.

Top Tip

Finding out your partner is pregnant is just as likely to dampen your libido as it is hers but you need to work through anything that may be stopping you, whether it's money worries, feeling freaked out by becoming a dad or feeling like you'd be pressuring her into having sex. You must not use any of these as an excuse not to have sex, even if your partner is making no advances or mention of the topic. She could be desperate for a bit of bedroom action but not be mentioning it to you for her own reasons.

The answer is simple. Talk about it. Come on, you are having a baby together so you should be able to talk about sex. Maybe broach the subject the next time you're watching television and a sex scene comes on, or when you're lying in bed together. A tentative advance may be enough to bring up the topic of conversation or – fingers crossed – solve the problem altogether.

TRAVEL

Upon finding out you are going to be a dad, it is probably too early to be buying anything baby-related. You may not want to tempt fate before you pass the important 12-week point when the risk of miscarriage drops dramatically. Plus it is way too early to find out whether you are having a boy or girl, so there's no point getting in the baby clothes just yet.

But there is one thing you should try to purchase if the budget allows: a holiday.

In about nine months' time, you are going to have near zero opportunity to go on a holiday where it is just the two of you for a good 18 years. This pregnancy is the last chance you and your partner will truly have to holiday together alone, where you can share a relaxing meal uninterrupted, laze by the pool uninterrupted and not have to go anywhere child-friendly.

So do your best to organise some sort of holiday, even if it is somewhere in the UK not too far away, or doing a house swap with friends. But if possible scrape together what you can to get away for a week abroad in the sunshine – ideally sometime during the early second trimester. You will earn mega brownie points if you suggest this to your partner and you will have a welcome distraction organising when and where to go.

Although you should start planning a trip now, the second trimester is the optimum time to travel by plane. In the first trimester, your partner will be suffering from nausea and tiredness which will making flying particularly unpleasant. In later pregnancy, it is just generally uncomfortable to be stuck on a plane for any length of time and after 28 weeks most airlines will want to see a letter from your midwife confirming the due date and that you are in good health and having a normal pregnancy. After 36 weeks your partner will not be allowed to fly (32 weeks for multiple births).

Regardless of when you are going, remember to help with the packing and other organising tasks where required and, of course, with the lifting of even slightly heavy luggage.

Top Tip

Unsurprisingly the moment your partner announces her pregnancy via social media and signs up to various baby-related websites, you are going to be bombarded with emails about all manner of baby products that marketing people will try to get you to buy. It's likely you will need none of it at this stage.

One such item I still to this day wish we had never purchased was a womb-listening device that enables you to hear your unborn baby more clearly by holding it to your partner's stomach and listening through headphones. Said device enabled you to speak to your baby via a microphone. It cost £50 back in 2006. Today a quick search on Amazon revealed similar devices ranging from £28 to £175 – the latter offers the chance for you to bring music to your unborn child in surround sound. What next – a plug-in device that makes your partner's womb viewable in HD?

Of course, it's up to you whether you think these are worthwhile purchases, but we used our device twice and both times it didn't work that well, if at all. For years it has been enough for parents to watch out for a first kick later in pregnancy and speak through cupped hands on the bump; does your unborn child really need a message coming over the womb tannoy saying: 'HELLO! IT'S YOUR DADDY HERE!'?

PETS AND PREGNANCY

If you own a pet, it is worth remembering that animals are potentially much more dangerous if you're pregnant.

The good news is that if you exercise care and common sense, then your pet will present no problems to your partner at all. Animals carry harmful parasites in their faeces and I see little point in scaremongering and listing them all here but suffice to say, some can be extremely harmful if passed on to your unborn baby.

Just make sure you are the one to pick up after your dog or change the litter tray – or if your partner has to do so, then she should wear disposable protective gloves (like the type you get in petrol stations) and wash her hands afterwards.

In fact washing your hands after any contact with an animal is a must. It is true an animal in the house will, over the long term, build up your – and your baby's – immune system but no need to take this theory too far.

The other thing to keep on top of is ensuring your cat and dog are regularly deflead. Once the baby arrives, flea bites may not be life-threatening but they will sure be unpleasant if the little one gets bitten. So best to sort the problem now.

Also if it is your partner who is particularly close to your dog, now is the time to start showing the dog more attention. When the baby comes along, your partner simply won't have as much time to devote to your dog, so getting him to develop relationships with others will help prepare him for changes to come.

Top Tip

If, like me, you own a big dog who likes jumping up at people, now is the time to train them out of such behaviour. Take them to a dog trainer if need be. You don't want them doing that to your partner when she is 35 weeks gone. A dog trainer may also help with preparing you to deal with issues that arise after the baby arrives and how your dog may react to the new addition.

CHAPTER 3
THE SECOND TRIMESTER: 13–27 WEEKS

So one trimester down, two to go. Congratulations! Mainly to your partner, obviously, but as the supportive other half, give yourself a tiny pat on the back too.

The good news is that the second trimester is considered by many mums to be the best. The risk of miscarriage has significantly reduced and your partner is beginning to get used to the idea that she is pregnant. At this stage, she can enjoy the positives of having a blossoming bump.

You will quite likely have made public the news of your forthcoming new arrival and you might even be having a few gatherings to celebrate. While you're partying, though, don't forget that all the while your baby is changing more than you could ever imagine…

FACTS ABOUT YOUR BABY'S DEVELOPMENT

A few weeks ago your baby was a cluster of cells, but now this amazing little thing has organs, nerves and muscles. She is beginning to sense things and how much she grows over the next three months will absolutely astound you.

▶ In **week 13**, your baby will start to pass urine. Tissue is also forming in her head and limbs which will form the basis of her skull and bones.

▶ Come **week 14**, your baby's arms will have reached the relative length that they'll be at birth. It is also around this time that the first signs appear of the baby's sex – a boy will be forming his prostate whilst a girl will be developing ovarian follicles. Alas, probably a little too early to detect on an ultrasound scan.

▶ The baby's scalp hair pattern will begin forming in **week 15**.

▶ In **week 16** the eyes are facing forward and beginning to move and the baby can make sucking motions. At around 11.5 cm from crown to rump, her movements are becoming more coordinated.

▶ Toenails appear around **week 17** and fat stores begin to form under the skin, ready to keep the baby warm after birth.

▶ Around **week 18** the ears may be sticking out and so your baby will start to hear things.

▶ Heard of vernix caseosa? It's this greasy cheese-like substance that forms around your baby's delicate skin in **week 19** to protect it from the abrasions and chapping that might otherwise happen through exposure to amniotic fluid. Just one small example of how incredible your unborn child is.

▶ Time to celebrate at **week 20** – this is the halfway point of a full-term pregnancy and you should be able to feel your baby moving by now.

▶ In **week 21** your baby will be able to swallow.

▸ In **week 22** her eyebrows could start showing.

▸ **Week 23** is a busy one – the baby's skin is becoming wrinkly and more translucent and fingerprints and footprints are forming. Meanwhile a boy's testes are descending from the abdomen and a girl's uterus and ovaries are in place complete with a lifetime's supply of eggs. Perhaps even more amazing is that it is possible for a baby to be born this week and survive with intensive medical care.

▸ By **week 24** your baby, now about 20 cm in length, is regularly sleeping and waking, whilst real hair will start growing on her head.

▸ In **week 25**, you can start having fun by seeing how your baby responds to your voice. Her startle reflexes and hands are developing so you should feel some movement when you speak to her through the tummy.

▸ It's the turn of the fingernails to appear in **week 26**. Meanwhile the lungs are producing a substance known as surfactant which allows the air sacs within the lungs to inflate and prevents them from sticking together when they deflate. In short, your baby is now equipped to breathe.

▸ **Week 27** marks the end of the second trimester and your baby's lungs and nervous system are continuing to mature. Some believe babies can dream at this stage. They certainly are prone to a spot of hiccups, which will be a strange but comforting sensation for your partner. By now the baby could be close to 25.5 cm long.

WHAT HAPPENS TO YOUR PARTNER'S BODY?

The good news is that after the thirteenth week your partner will probably feel less nauseous, less tired and less in need of the toilet (though not for long). Sometimes she may not even feel pregnant at all – although the growing bump as the womb expands and moves upwards will make sure she doesn't truly forget.

Here is a rundown of the main things that happen to her body in the second trimester:

▶ **Between 13 and 18 weeks**, your partner may start getting a few spots as hormonal changes begin to affect her skin. There may be small changes in pigmentation, where it looks darker in places. Meanwhile, a dark line might appear from her navel down the centre of her abdomen. This is called the linea nigra, which will fade after birth. Now's the time to stock up on moisturiser for her to use to prevent stretch marks.

▶ Around **week 19** your partner's uterus will start pushing into her abdomen and onto her diaphragm so she will begin to feel breathless more quickly. If you're out and about on foot, make sure she is taking regular breaks. Embrace elevators and avoid even slightly hilly routes. And, don't forget, as the baby grows and begins to press down on the bladder, the need for her to make more frequent trips to the toilet will return!

▶ You'll be able to feel the baby from this point on, but by **week 24** the kicking and moving about will be fairly persistent (a hint at life to come!) and your partner will be feeling like a punchbag, as well as being achy and uncomfortable with all the extra weight.

Top Tip Always be mindful of how cumbersome and uncomfortable it is for your partner to be carrying your baby 24/7. As my 27-weeks-pregnant wife put it when, late one evening, I dared to suggest that we walk the seven-minute walk home from the bus stop, 'You try doing it with a couple of coconuts and a giant watermelon strapped to your chest.' There wasn't a lot I could say to that, really, other than hail a taxi.

DEALING WITH SECOND TRIMESTER HEALTH CONDITIONS

At this stage of pregnancy, your partner (and you) would have learnt to deal with a lot of the symptoms encountered in the first trimester and hopefully by now some of them, like morning sickness, will have eased.

Here are some new symptoms that she is most likely to encounter in the second trimester and, once again, how you can help her deal with them:

BRAXTON HICKS CONTRACTIONS

What on earth are these? You'd have probably heard the phrase mentioned in your partner's conversations with other pregnant women but don't worry – they are extremely common! John Braxton Hicks was the name of the doctor who first noticed that pregnant women were having contractions well before they were due to give birth.

Hopefully you'll know what contractions are – or at least that they are synonymous with labour pains, so why on earth are they cropping up now? Well, it is your partner's uterus preparing for the big job ahead – 'warm-ups' that your partner will feel in her abdomen at unpredictable moments. They will have actually started around the sixth week of pregnancy but only now will your partner start to feel them. That said, not all pregnant women will feel them so don't be alarmed if that is the case.

What should I do? The contractions are almost always nothing to worry about and your partner may not even mention them. But in the rare instance where they become painful and regular, it could be a sign of pre-term labour and you should contact your midwife immediately. Exercise is thought to help ease Braxton Hicks contractions – if it doesn't, it could well be a sign of actual labour.

When do they stop? For those who experience them, these contractions will continue into the third trimester by which time the irregular, infrequent cramping will become strong, frequent cramping and then finally actual labour pains.

NASAL PROBLEMS

Why? Pregnancy increases the circulation and therefore more blood flows through your partner's mucous membranes. This causes the lining of her nostrils to swell, restricting airflow and possibly causing snoring, congestion and even nosebleeds.

What should I do? Again, the good old-fashioned ways to clear a blocked nose may suffice. There's nothing particularly romantic about bringing your partner a bowl of hot water and a towel to cover her head so why not run her a warm bath instead? Decongestants shouldn't be taken during pregnancy but a pharmacist might be able to recommend an appropriate nasal spray that doesn't contain any. If it is really causing your partner a problem, her GP may be able to prescribe antihistamines.

When will it stop? After birth.

LEG CRAMPS

Why? There is no firm answer for this. Experts put the sensation down to anything from the body struggling to deal with the increase in blood circulation to the increased pressure that the growing baby puts on nerve endings and blood vessels. It may also be because the legs are getting tired carrying around the extra weight and then cramping when resting. Leg cramps – which occur in the calf muscles – can become more painful and frequent mid pregnancy (around the 20-week mark), to the point that they might wake her up in the middle of the night. Though they last up to ten minutes, they will not do any long-term damage to her calf muscles.

What should I do? Luckily there is quite a lot you can do, other than just sympathise. When they strike, get your partner to straighten her leg, beginning with the foot, and gently flex her ankle and toes – this will hurt at first but the pain will ease. Then you can massage the cramped muscle. After that if she walks around for a few minutes on her heels, the cramp should pass, though the muscle may be sore and tender for up to 24 hours.

To prevent further cramps, you can encourage her to do some daily foot exercises and calf stretches to help prevent them (see below). Before bed, you could also run her a warm bath (but not hot as hot baths can damage the baby's cells) and use a pillow or wedge at the bottom of the bed for her to prop her feet on and to keep the duvet loose during the night. Drinking plenty of water throughout the day may also help.

In very rare cases, leg cramps could indicate a blood clot. Call your GP if the cramp is constant, if there is swelling and tenderness around the affected muscle and if this tender area feels warm and looks red.

When will they stop? They tend to get worse and more common in the third trimester, when around a third of pregnant women tend to suffer from cramp.

Exercises to prevent leg cramps

There are two exercises that, carried out daily, could stave off the cramps.

▶ **Calf stretches** – your partner should stand about a metre from a wall, lean forward and stretch her arms so she touches the wall. Keep the feet flat on the floor. Hold for five seconds. Repeat for five minutes, three times a day, ideally once before going to bed.

▶ **Foot exercises** – your partner should stretch and bend each foot up and down quickly 30 times. Then rotate each foot eight times one way, then eight times the other.

BLADDER AND KIDNEY INFECTIONS

Why? With the uterus expanding and hormonal changes slowing the flow of urine from the kidney to the bladder, the risk of bladder and kidney infections increases.

What should I do? Don't underestimate the potential threat these infections pose. A urinary tract infection (or cystitis) could irritate your partner's womb into labour, meaning the baby is born too soon. Quick antibiotic treatment is vital. Look out for these signs:

▶ She has pain in the lower tummy or back that may feel like contractions

▶ She finds it painful to pass water

▶ She has blood in the urine

▶ She is weeing even more than usual

▶ She is generally feeling unwell

If these occur, then she should call the midwife. If the infection has spread to her kidneys, then it is even more serious. Go to A & E immediately if she experiences the following:

▶ A temperature of 38°C or higher

▶ Severe pain in back, pelvis or side

▶ Shaking and shivering

▶ Nausea and vomiting

▶ Diarrhoea

When will they stop? The risk of your partner developing a kidney infection is extremely small (just 1 in 830 pregnant women do) but

1 in 10 develop some sort of urinary infection so remain vigilant throughout the whole pregnancy.

VAGINAL BLEEDING

Why? Vaginal bleeding or spotting is actually quite common in early and mid-term pregnancy. There can be numerous causes and most are harmless and no cause for concern. But that won't stop you worrying about the rare cases where it indicates something more serious such as miscarriage or an ectopic pregnancy. But, rest assured, by the second trimester, the risk of these have significantly reduced and vaginal bleeding may be an indication of:

▸ irritation to the uterus (such as through having sex)

▸ fibroids on the uterine wall

▸ cervical polyp

▸ cervical or vaginal infection

▸ an inherited blood disorder such as Von Willebrand disease, that may be making it more difficult for your partner's blood to clot

▸ later on in the second trimester, it might be an indication of placenta praevia, where the placenta is resting at the bottom of the uterus between the baby and the cervix

Rest assured, if treated, all of these conditions pose no risk to your baby at all. Some may not even require treatment if they are not causing too much discomfort and as long as there are no other symptoms.

What should I do? Book an appointment with the GP or midwife to put your minds at rest as soon as possible.

When will it stop? If treated, then it should stop occurring but if it continues to persist, do not hesitate to seek further medical help.

PRE-ECLAMPSIA

Pre-eclampsia is a condition of pregnancy that is characterised by high blood pressure and high protein levels in the urine. No one knows what causes it but it is believed to arise from problems with the placenta, which connects your partner's blood supply to the baby's organs. It usually occurs in the third trimester but can develop any time after 20 weeks. Around six per cent of pregnant women will be affected by some form of mild pre-eclampsia, whilst just 1–2 per cent will develop more severe cases of the condition. So it is rare but you should be on regular alert for symptoms because left untreated, pre-eclampsia could lead to your partner suffering liver or kidney failure, seizures, a stroke and even brain damage, whilst it could lead to your baby being born prematurely or even stillborn.

It is estimated that approximately 1,000 babies a year die in the UK as a result of pre-eclampsia but it is very much treatable. The earlier pre-eclampsia is diagnosed and monitored, the better the outlook for mother and baby.

Symptoms of pre-eclampsia

High blood pressure and high protein levels in the urine are difficult things to detect without being tested so be on your guard if any of the following develop:

▶ Swelling of the feet, ankles, face or hands – or any excessive weight gain – caused by water retention (oedema)

▶ Severe headache

▶ Vision problems, such as blurriness or seeing flashing lights

▶ Severe heartburn

▶ Pain below the ribs

▶ Nausea or vomiting

If your partner suffers from any of these, she should seek medical advice immediately.

Another sign of pre-eclampsia comes from the baby. If she is growing more slowly than she should be, then this suggests a reduction in nutrients and oxygen being passed from mother to baby, caused by a limited blood supply through the placenta. If this is the case, it will soon be picked up at one of your antenatal appointments when the midwife or doctor measures the baby.

Is my partner at risk of pre-eclampsia?

Studies have shown that your partner is more at risk, and therefore you should be even more vigilant for the symptoms of pre-eclampsia, if:

▶ she has an existing medical condition such as diabetes, kidney disease, high blood pressure, Hughes syndrome (or an increased risk of blood clotting) or lupus

▶ she has suffered with pre-eclampsia in a previous pregnancy

Furthermore there is a small increased risk if two of the following apply to her:

▶ It's her first pregnancy

▶ She was last pregnant over ten years ago

▶ She has a family history of the condition

▶ She's over 40

▶ Her BMI at the start of pregnancy was 35 or over

▶ She's having a multiple birth

It is likely that a midwife would have picked up these risks sooner and will have advised your partner to take 75 mg of aspirin per day from 12 weeks until the baby is born. Evidence suggests this lowers the chances of developing pre-eclampsia.

How is pre-eclampsia treated?

Pre-eclampsia can only be cured by delivering the baby. If your partner is diagnosed with the condition, then she will be closely monitored until it is safe for the baby to be born – usually around 37 or 38 weeks. Upon diagnosis, your partner will be referred to a hospital specialist for further assessment and treatment where necessary.

If her only symptom is high blood pressure and there are no other signs of pre-eclampsia, then it should be possible for her to go home and attend regular follow-up appointments, which could well be daily.

But if there are other signs, then your partner will have to be admitted to hospital until the baby can be delivered. Her blood pressure and urine can be tested regularly and also she may have regular ultrasound scans to ensure blood is flowing through the placenta and that the baby is growing as she should be. The baby's breathing and movements can also be properly observed this way and additionally the baby's heart rate may be monitored to detect any sign of stress or distress.

What if my partner is admitted to hospital with pre-eclampsia?

Rest assured, your partner and baby will be in good hands with medical staff on standby to deal with any complications that arise from pre-eclampsia. However, the thought of having to be in hospital until the birth will not be a pleasant one for your partner and your job now will be to make her extended stay as comfortable and worry-free as possible. It is worth bearing in mind the following:

▶ Make sure she has a mobile phone and a tablet/laptop to keep her entertained and in touch with people, along with all the relevant chargers.

▶ Make sure she has what she needs in terms of toiletries and make-up to help her feel at home. Get a list of items from her.

▶ Make sure she is regularly supplied with clean laundry, whether you do it yourself or enlist the help of another reliable relative.

▶ Bring in cushions and other small items that will remind her of home. A few photographs might be nice too.

▶ Your partner's place of work will need to be informed and she will probably make first contact here, but do whatever she requests to ensure her work worries are kept at an absolute minimum.

▶ Of course, you'll be unlikely to be able to take much time off your work to keep her company but do your best to ring her during the day and obviously go and visit her after work and at weekends.

▶ Bring her tasty healthy snacks. A decent flask of (decaff) tea or coffee will go down well – and save money.

▶ Bring her items such as magazines, newspapers and puzzle books to help pass the time.

▶ Keep the baby plans on track in terms of things that you need to buy and do. Looking on the bright side, the enforced hospital stay will actually give you a chance to make more of the decisions together and get you involved.

▶ Intimate contact will be nigh on impossible now so don't be shy about simple things like holding her hand and stroking her hair as you spend time together. It is a really difficult time, perhaps the worst time for someone to have to stay in hospital, so do not allow it to come between you. Instead strengthen the bond by doing all that you can to make it easier and stress-free for her. This will be good for the baby too.

ANTENATAL CARE

By now your midwife will have determined whether your partner needs extra care throughout the pregnancy to check that she and the baby are both well – i.e. if she has an increased risk of developing a certain condition such as pre-eclampsia. In most cases, however, you can expect this steady trickle of antenatal appointments throughout the second trimester:

THE 16-WEEK APPOINTMENT

What's it for? To arrange the next ultrasound scan and check that everything is fine with the baby and for your partner to air any concerns or ask any questions that she may have.

What will it tell us? Your partner will have her blood pressure checked and urine tested to ensure protein levels are normal. Any other screening tests she might need will be reviewed, discussed and recorded. Generally, anything that is likely to cause any problems for your partner and the baby will be picked up here.

Should I be there? Not really. The appointment should be quick, though have your mobile phone to hand just in case there are any problems arising or just so she can give you a progress report afterwards and let you know all is well.

THE ANOMALY SCAN

When? Between 18 and 20 weeks.

What's it for? The main purpose of this appointment is for a sonographer to check the physical development of your baby. They will look at where the placenta is lying in the uterus.

What will it tell us? The scan will point out if there are any physical abnormalities with your baby. The sonographer will give you a guided tour of your baby, pointing out the face and hands, and measure parts of the body such as head circumference, abdominal circumference, spine and thigh bone to check that they all match up with the sizes expected, according to the due date. They will also check that the baby's heart and kidneys are working properly. In short, it is a full service and if there are any issues, you will be told straight away and a midwife or doctor will be consulted for further analysis and advice. Don't worry if your sonographer needs to conduct a repeat scan – this happens in about 15 per cent of cases and doesn't mean anything is wrong, rather that the baby is in an awkward position and the sonographer cannot see everything that they need to see.

And perhaps most exciting of all, this is the scan where you can find out – if you wish – the sex of the baby.

Should I be there? Yes. For a start the detailed scan is another moment not to be missed, but also, in the event of there being any issues, you will be a much needed hand for your partner to hold and also the midwife and doctor might want to ask you questions about your family medical history. Oh, and that moment when you find out if you are having a boy or a girl is another memory to treasure.

THE 25-WEEK APPOINTMENT

After this, if this is your partner's first pregnancy, then she will be invited for another appointment towards the end of the second trimester, at around 25 weeks. A midwife or doctor will measure the size of her uterus and also check her blood pressure and test her urine to check her protein levels. One of the things they will want to assess is the risk of your partner developing pre-eclampsia. If the baby is smaller than she should be, then your partner will be invited back for more scans to monitor growth carefully.

Top Tip

Should we find out the baby's sex? If I am being honest, I had to go back and add in this bit about finding out the sex of your baby at the anomaly scan. Why? Well, to me, it's a no-brainer – why wouldn't you want to find out? What is the significance of waiting until the baby is born? It's a baby already and knowing if it's a boy or a girl helps you to organise and plan, even if it is just getting the right colour scheme in the nursery. However, I accept that people will want to keep it as a surprise, but you must agree as a couple whether or not you are going to want to find out the baby's sex at the scan.

FOODS TO EAT AND FOODS TO AVOID

This list doesn't vary greatly from the one for the first trimester but it is a good idea to up your intake slightly of wholegrain fibre and fruit and vegetables, and ensure you are getting good helpings of calcium and protein and omega-3 fats – without significantly increasing your intake of sugars and saturated fats.

Simple meals and snacks to help your partner to do this include:

- A quality fruit and nut muesli (not the powdery Swiss-style bird food variety) topped with bananas and berries, then low-fat natural yoghurt and a spoonful of honey

- Wholegrain pizzas topped with vegetables, with a good helping of low-fat pasteurised cheese

- Lentil-based vegetable soup – it's easy to knock up a batch to last a couple of days

- Raw vegetables such as cucumber, peppers, carrots and even broccoli, with yoghurt-based dips

- Try branching out in the fruit and veg aisle to avoid boredom – swap green beans for sweet potatoes and apples and pears for mangoes and pineapple

- Have cooked (preferably steamed or poached) white fish such as cod or haddock at least twice a week for those omega-3 fats. Alternatively, if your partner really doesn't like seafood, get her to snack on walnuts, kiwi fruit or flaxseeds.

ALCOHOL

By now your partner knows she is pregnant and so the consumption of any alcohol must be discouraged. However, there is no harm in occasionally indulging in alcohol-free lager. Avoid too much reliance on no-alcohol fruit punches as the sugar content is usually very high.

TRAVEL

By now you will have booked your second trimester trip away and you will be raring to go. It is a perfect time to travel as morning sickness and nausea will hopefully have passed and restrictions on air travel don't usually come into force until the third trimester, but it is worth taking the following precautions:

▶ Keep moving to prevent blood clots – whether you are travelling by train, plane or car, your partner should keep her circulation moving. She should wiggle or massage her legs every few minutes and get up to walk around at least once an hour – so this entails regular stops whilst driving longer distances and bagging an aisle seat on the plane or train. If she can prop up her feet, all the better.

▶ Get in plenty of bottled water so your partner doesn't get dehydrated or tired – stock up beforehand for train journeys and car journeys to avoid overpriced buffet cars and service stations.

▶ This is how she should fasten her seatbelt safely:

1. Strap the lap section of the belt across her thighs and under her bump, not across it (as the pressure across the belly could cause damage).

2. The diagonal shoulder section should go across her collarbone, between her breasts.

3. Fasten it so that it sits above the bump, not over it.

▶ Get her comfy – don't forget to pack a back-support cushion or pillow to prevent cramp.

▶ For a smoother ride, get seats on the front half of the plane.

Top Tip

One weekend while my partner went away, I held a paint party with the lads to help spruce up the baby's nursery. Some were dads and made sure we got in low-fume, child-friendly paints and floor covering. We got the whole thing done in a day and it only cost me a few beers. My partner was thrilled when she got back – especially as one of the lads had also donated a cot they no longer needed.

EXERCISE

There is no reason your partner shouldn't continue exercising based on the considerations and stipulations of exercising in the first trimester. It will keep up her energy levels and help her sleep at night. At this stage it is still safe to exercise daily, so long as she responds appropriately to any warning signals that her body gives her to stop. These include:

- ▶ Dizziness or light-headedness

- ▶ Headache

- ▶ Fatigue

- ▶ Nausea and vomiting

- ▶ Dehydration or overheating

- ▶ Pain in the lower back or stomach

- ▶ Unusual vaginal discharge or bleeding

It's fine to continue with a mixture of aerobic exercise such as swimming or walking and strength-building exercises such as light stretches. It is important to be mindful of the following:

▶ After 16 weeks, your partner shouldn't exercise by lying on her back. Apart from being uncomfortable, this position means the uterus puts weight on a major blood vessel known as the vena cava, which may restrict blood flow to the baby and to your partner's brain, causing dizziness. She should prop herself up on her elbows or lean on her left side.

▶ As the pregnancy progresses, your partner's body produces a hormone called relaxin, which does what it sounds like. It's responsible for loosening joints in preparation for a growing baby, meaning your partner will be more susceptible to sprains, so towards the end of this trimester, she should be avoiding high-energy aerobic exercise and excessive stretching.

▶ The increased weight will adjust your partner's centre of gravity and she will lose her balance more easily – another reason to avoid high-energy aerobic exercise.

▶ Like with any exercising at any time, it is important to warm up and wind down appropriately so there are no surprises for the heart rate.

SEX

We established in the first trimester that pregnancy is actually a good time for couples to have sex, and now in the second trimester, as the nausea and morning sickness hopefully eases and your partner grows more comfortable with her new shape, there is a good chance that her libido will increase. Pregnancy hormones will also be making her skin glow and her hair shinier – this is the classic 'blooming' stage that others sometimes notice and it's likely you will too.

You may fret that her growing bump is getting in the way, or it will make her uncomfortable, but why not try out some – or all – of the following positions and see which ones work for you both:

▶ **Woman on top** – if your partner gets to straddle you, it will take the pressure off her back and belly and enable her to control the depth of the thrusting. Plus, well, what a view for you!

▶ **Sitting** – you sit in an armless chair and your partner faces and straddles you. It's extremely intimate as you can look one another in the eye. Aw.

▶ **Side by side** – lying side by side, facing one another will again allow your partner to rest her belly and you will both enjoy the intimacy and gentleness, although towards the end of the second trimester, the bump will, I am afraid, make it tricky for you to reach.

▶ **Spooning** – similar to side by side but you lie behind your partner and enjoy a lovely cuddle while you are having sex. The position avoids deep penetration which will prove uncomfortable for your partner as the third trimester approaches.

▶ **Hands and knees** – also known as 'doggy style', this is where your partner rests on her hands and knees and you enter her from behind. But for comfort, place some pillows underneath her to support her belly and breasts.

Top Tip

If you are having your first baby, this is the last time you will truly have together as a couple while looking this young and this sexy. No, really – it cannot be stressed enough how much the two of you should embrace this time of your lives before the onslaught of tiredness, dirty nappies and constant baby talk takes over. Arrange a few date nights in where you just come home and enjoy a nice (easy to prepare) meal and early night together. And make sure you have the odd lazy weekend where you shut off the outside world and spend as much of it in bed as possible.

PATERNITY LEAVE AND PAY

Once you know the due date, it is advisable to give yourself time to think about what you want to take in the way of paternity leave.

What am I entitled to? If you earn over £112 per week, then you are entitled to Statutory Paternity Pay. BUT you have to have been working in your current job for at least 26 weeks continuously when your partner is 15 weeks gone (known as the 'qualifying week'). Current Statutory Paternity Pay is £139.58 per week or 90 per cent of your average weekly earnings (whichever is lower) but check the latest HMRC figures here: www.gov.uk/paternity-pay-leave/overview. Usually you will be eligible for one to two weeks' paternity pay but if you're planning to be a full-time carer to your baby while your partner is returning to work in the baby's first year and stopping her maternity pay entitlement, then you may be entitled to Statutory Shared Parental Pay (see below). Again, check the HMRC website.

What about time off? In addition to this paid time off, you are entitled to take a further 18 weeks of unpaid paternity leave – again, you have to have been working in your job for at least 26 weeks continuously come the qualifying week.

What if I haven't been there that long? If this doesn't apply to you, book off the required time as holiday and remember that you are entitled to take this paternity leave (unpaid, remember) at any time up until when your child turns 18.

So how much should I take? This will depend on financial considerations and also on your partner's circumstances. The best thing to do is to find out what you are entitled to in terms of pay – both from the government and your employer – and start doing your sums. You may have some sort of paid paternity leave incentive with your job, especially if you have been there for some time, but there's a good chance that your partner will have the better deal that will last for longer (sometimes up to a year, often at a percentage of salary for the last six months) – again, especially if she has been working there for a long time. In any case, your partner doesn't need to have been working for any minimum period to be entitled to Statutory Maternity Leave (39 weeks paid). Sadly many of us do not have the luxury of having both mum and dad off for an extended period on a reduced income, and the typical amount of time that new dads take off is two weeks from the birth date. Having said that, if your partner is the higher earner, then she may want to return to work sooner and hand the day care baton to you, in which case you may be entitled to Statutory Shared Parental Pay, so long as she is no longer claiming any kind of maternity benefit.

When do I need to decide? There's no pressure. You must just give your employer at least three weeks' notice in advance of the due date as to the length of time you intend to take off initially. Nothing is set in stone – you'll be entitled to leave earlier if the baby arrives earlier or later or if you need to extend your period of time off if, for instance, your partner is recovering from having a Caesarean. So what are you waiting for – let them know tomorrow and do the maths later. You may have to inform them in writing rather than just by email so check if this is the case.

> **Top Tip**
>
> Still to decide or agree on a name? Make a nice date night of it and see if you can nail one you like. Get in some nice food, put on some music and just sit and talk it out. Or go on a day out somewhere and keep it on the conversation agenda. Turn the decision process into real together time rather than a last-minute hasty choice in the maternity unit!

THINGS TO BUY

Now that you have passed the first trimester, you will do well to think ahead and start deciding what you need to buy for the baby, perhaps budgeting to spend a certain amount every month so the inevitable bills don't come as too much of a shock to the bank account!

It's quite likely that your partner will have already been checking out various products in baby magazines and catalogues but a good first step is to see just what you can source from elsewhere, i.e. if you or your partner have a sibling or friends with older children who have no need for all the baby paraphernalia that is clogging up their attic.

Potentially you could save hundreds and hundreds of pounds by accepting such generosity – so long as you adhere to the following rules of thumb:

▶ Don't be polite – only take what you need, rather than acting as a house clearance service for your well-meaning relative or friend. Otherwise you will end up with a home full of someone else's clutter whilst still having to buy whatever the item was that you wanted in the first place.

▶ Try not to be put off by the way things look – if something is a bit old-fashioned but still works, then great.

▶ Second-hand items can usually scrub up well, so long as they are still in good working order. But don't use second-hand Moses baskets and cot mattresses because these increase the risk of cot death. Also avoid second-hand baby car seats as you cannot be sure that they have never been in a crash or suffered wear and tear that deem their protective power ineffective.

▶ Welcome baby clothes with open arms. In the first year of a baby's life, you will never have too many sleepsuits.

▶ Check that flat-pack cots have all the required pieces before taking. If you are not confident enough to substitute a missing screw or bar in a baby-safe manner, then acquire elsewhere or buy something new.

Top Tip

Ask for an inventory of just what might be available for you to take and what you will need in the way of a vehicle to transport it all home. Don't make the mistake I did and hire a van to drive up from London to Northumberland, only to return with barely enough to fill the boot of a Nissan Micra.

TO BUY OR NOT TO BUY

So what should you consider buying new, if your relatives or friends don't have anything you require in stock? It is clearly worth making a list to help you budget but here are a few things worth bearing in mind about certain items before you make that commitment to buy:

▶ **Moses basket** – though it may seem a superfluous purchase in that your baby will very quickly outgrow it and you may even find that you mostly bypass the basket and put him down to sleep in a cot, it does allow the flexibility and portability for a sleeping baby to be carried from room to room in the first few weeks.

▶ **Baby sleeping bag** – when your new baby arrives, you will spend weeks trying to perfect the swaddling technique with a good old-fashioned blanket, as a matter of principle. And yet, invest in a few of these (making sure they are the correct tog for the season, as you would a duvet), and you'll see it's far simpler to slip the baby into one and fasten accordingly.

▶ **Changing bag** – this is absolutely essential to help you get out and about and be on the move with your baby, and as dad-to-be, you'd do well to get involved with the purchasing of one so you are as happy to carry the thing about with you as your partner will be. Once purchased, help stock it up with nappies and wipes and nappy cream and nappy bags so you know EXACTLY where everything is when you suddenly find yourself alone with your yowling baby in a supermarket baby changing room, conscious of the queue of mums and dads waiting outside to change their little ones.

▶ **Changing table** – this serves as a place at home to store everything you need for changing the baby from the mat resting on the top to all the wipes, nappies, cream and bags stored neatly underneath. I considered it an unnecessary luxury at first but quickly realised it was a real help for establishing a routine for parent and baby.

▶ **Cot** – if you are buying a new one, it may be worth considering the future. A cot that converts into a bed at toddler stage might cost more now but will save the expense and hassle of having to buy a toddler bed a year or so down the line. Don't put it too near a window and certainly not by a radiator – and make sure you don't use a second-hand cot mattress, since, as mentioned earlier, this increases the risk of cot death.

▶ **Newborn baby bath supports** – as first-time parents, you are going to bathe the baby with utmost caution and there are various types of bath supports available that can be used with a baby bath or in your main bath to keep your baby safe.

▶ **Blackout blinds** – good for the baby's room to block out all the light at nap time and will stop him waking too early in the summer months once he is sleeping through the night. Ensure blinds are cordless to avoid entanglement.

▶ **Car seat** – another purchase worth giving yourself some time to work out how to use and display the utmost confidence in doing so. If you have a car with Isofix fittings, you are already at an advantage because it is perhaps the easiest – and a very safe – car seat locking system. In fact if you are in the process of changing cars to accommodate the new addition, make sure your new car has this. Then it is just a case of working out how to put the baby in safely. Pick a seat you are happy with and then practise, practise, practise, remembering that until the baby weighs at least 9 kg, the seat should be placed in the car rear-facing.

▶ **Baby buggy** – you're looking for one that folds down flat nice and easily (a one-click-and-fold mechanism is ideal) and also one that is lightweight to carry about, yet sturdy. It is definitely worth going to a baby store showroom to test a few models. Then, as with the car seat, practise folding it up and away. Again, you might want to think ahead and purchase a buggy that can go on to accommodate a baby and a toddler for when your baby gets older and you're thinking of having another.

THE BIRTH PLAN

What is it? The plan's main purpose is for your partner to communicate her wishes to the midwife and doctor. The factors that a birth plan may consider include:

- ▶ **Birth partner** – i.e. the person she wants to be present at the birth (hopefully, you)

- ▶ **Positions for the birth** – anything from being propped up on all fours with pillows, or using birthing balls or beanbags, or if she wants to use a birthing pool and give birth in water. It's fine for the baby – the placenta is the ultimate scuba diving equipment.

- ▶ **Pain relief** – such as epidurals or gas and air. See below.

- ▶ **Having a Caesarean** – depending on preference and medical advice. Again, see below.

- ▶ **Having a home birth**

- ▶ **What intervention is welcome** – e.g. in certain circumstances where it might be helpful, medication to speed up birth or a preference to use forceps

- ▶ **Placenta delivery** – after the baby is born, the placenta needs to be delivered. This is usually induced by an injection of oxytocic medicine in the thigh to bring on contractions. Your partner can request to deliver it naturally instead.

Should I get involved? To an extent, but mainly in the capacity of listening to what your partner wants and being ready to act on any parts that you may be able to help with, such as remembering to bring a favourite cushion from home or playing suitable music. It is also a good opportunity for you to familiarise yourself with the childbirth process so you are as clued up as possible.

When should I object? In most cases you should leave all the decisions to your partner and only advise, but you may have certain opinions that you wish to express and for your partner to consider. For instance, if you feel strongly about not having a home birth, then say so.

How do I ensure the plan is implemented? Your partner will give the plan to her midwife but it is important for you to have a copy too, so you can study it and refer to it during labour.

PAIN RELIEF: THE OPTIONS

Though it is not your place to decide on the types of pain relief that your partner uses during childbirth, it is, of course, helpful for you to know the various options available to her so you can be clear on what each one entails.

- ▶ **Entonox (gas and air)** – this is a mixture of oxygen and nitrous oxide gas. It doesn't stop the pain but eases it and many women opt for it because it is easy to use and they can control it themselves. Plus it is totally safe for the baby.

- ▶ **Intramuscular injection** – this is an injection of pethidine or diamorphine in the buttock or thigh muscle. It can be administered by a midwife straight away and takes 20 minutes to work, lasting between two and four hours. It will help your partner to relax without slowing down the labour. It can make it more difficult to push and if given too close to delivery, it can affect the baby's breathing, but in that case, another drug will be administered to reverse the effects.

▸ **Epidural** – by far the most effective and very commonly used these days. It is a local anaesthetic – and hence needs to be administered by an anaesthetist – that numbs the nerves that carry the pain impulses from the birth canal to the brain. In most cases it gives complete pain relief, especially welcome if a woman is experiencing a long labour or is in distress. Bear in mind, some epidural anaesthetics can numb the legs, making your partner less mobile immediately after the birth (meaning an overnight stay in hospital), or leave her with a headache or backache for a day or two but overall it is considered a safe method for both mother and baby, with the risk of permanent damage to the mother being anything between 1 in 80,000 and 1 in 320,000, according to the NHS. The best thing for your partner to do is to research what an epidural entails and discuss any concerns or questions with the midwife.

▸ **Alternative therapies** such as acupuncture, aromatherapy, homeopathy, hypnosis, massage and reflexology may offer some pain relief, though this is mostly unproven. You will have to make provision for these as the NHS will not have the resources to provide them.

▸ **Some methods of birth** are designed to ease pain relief naturally, such as giving birth in a birthing pool so the water can ease the pain of contractions.

THE C-WORD: CAESAREAN

What is it? A Caesarean birth is an operation to deliver the baby through a surgical incision in the mother's abdomen and uterus. In some circumstances it is scheduled in advance, for the reasons given below (among others), and if any apply the midwife will discuss this option with your partner ahead of the due date. In others it is carried out in response to an unforeseen complication – for more information on emergency Caesareans, see p.136 in Chapter 5.

When will she need one? Usually there has to be a medical reason as to why one is given, although your partner can choose to have one so long as her obstetrician agrees. Sometimes she may be referred to another who may approve or, if she is choosing to have one because she is anxious about the birth, she may be referred to a healthcare professional with expertise in helping her confront and deal with her anxiety. Alternatively she may be required to go for an emergency Caesarean during the labour where circumstances suggest she should have one – again, for more on this see p.136 in Chapter 5.

Common reasons for a woman to undergo a scheduled Caesarean include – but are not limited to – the following:

▶ She develops severe pre-eclampsia

▶ She's had two or more Caesarean sections

▶ She has a small pelvis

▶ She is having a multiple birth

▶ The baby is in an awkward position, i.e. with the bottom or feet rather than the head nearest the pelvis (breeched)

▶ She has a medical condition that may put her at risk during labour, such as a heart condition

▶ She develops a viral infection such as herpes

▶ She has placenta praevia (when the placenta blocks the entrance to the womb)

▶ The baby's growth is restricted – some babies who are not growing well in the womb have a higher risk of being ill or dying around the time of birth

▶ Women over 35 are more likely to need a Caesarean because they are more at risk from conditions such as gestational diabetes, slow widening of the cervix and high blood pressure.

Is it a risky operation? All surgical procedures involve a certain amount of risk and the following may develop:

▶ Infection of the womb lining and the wound itself – though nowadays the practice is to administer antibiotics before operating to minimise this outcome

▶ Blood clot (thrombosis) in the legs which is dangerous if the clot breaks off and lodges in the lungs

▶ Damage to the bladder or ureter

▶ Excess bleeding

Rest assured, it is still very rare for women who have had a Caesarean to end up in an intensive care unit. If your partner thinks a scheduled

Caesarean might be the best choice, she should do her own research on the procedure and speak to the medical professionals at every opportunity.

Should I get involved with the decision? Not really, beyond supporting her in her choice. A Caesarean section is a very common procedure these days so there is no need to worry. Afterwards your partner will be able to stay in hospital for up to four days and it takes about six weeks to heal completely. In that time she will be able to look after her baby and herself as normal, so long as she takes a few precautions such as avoiding climbing stairs too often and not driving.

SHOULD WE HAVE A HOME BIRTH?

The thought of being able to give birth in your own familiar surroundings and the baby's first experience of the outside world being its new home is reason enough for any pregnant woman to consider a home birth. But as natural as it sounds, it does involve a great deal of careful thought.

First and foremost, discuss your wish for a home birth with your midwife or doctor. If your partner has a medical condition that might cause complications during labour or if she has a history of difficult births or has suffered a miscarriage in the past, it is likely that they will recommend a hospital birth. It's also the case if you live some distance from a hospital. It's important to note that pain relief options are limited for home births – for instance, you need to be in a hospital to have an epidural.

If all is well, then you will probably be allocated a community midwife who, when your partner is in labour, will come out and assess her and see how she is coping. If your partner is in early labour, then the midwife may leave and come back later. Whatever happens they will return with another midwife so there are two present as your partner is giving birth. This means one of them can look after your partner and the other can take care of the baby. It is highly likely that a midwife would stay with you throughout the whole labour for a first pregnancy but this may be one of the things that you should check.

If you do opt for a home birth initially, you are fine to change your minds later and have the baby in a hospital or birth centre.

YOUR OWN PLAN FOR THE BIRTH

Whilst your partner is formulating her birth plan, it is probably a good time to make firm decisions as to what you want to do at the birth, with her blessing that is. The two big questions are:

1. **Do I watch the baby come out?** Many men might shiver at the very thought, while others will already be picking which camera lens they are going to have ready for the big entrance. Decide now so at the birth when the midwife asks if you want to see the little one at the crucial moment, you are not there umming and aahing or rubbing your chin going, 'Ooh, should I?' – you can just say 'OK' or 'Oh, no thanks, I'm fine here.' It's best to discuss this with your partner.

2. **Do I cut the cord?** Again, decide now. Many men opt to do this so they feel they have played an important part in the birth. It takes a matter of moments and then you can return to your partner's side so that you can welcome your new addition together.

CHAPTER 4
THE THIRD TRIMESTER: 28–40 WEEKS

There was probably a moment when your partner first fell pregnant that you thought you had ages before you would actually be a parent, holding a baby in your arms. Nine months? Pah! That's practically an eon. It's plenty of time to contemplate the reality of fatherhood, right?

Not so, I'm afraid. Here you are in the third and final trimester and be in no doubt – the last few weeks of your partner's pregnancy will fly by and before you know it, you'll be a dad. If the thought of all that responsibility still makes you feel uneasy and unprepared, you will have a chance to practise by doing your best to look after your partner as labour day approaches.

Of course, your unease is nothing compared to hers. These last few weeks are extremely hard for her. By now she's most probably tired of being pregnant.

More than likely, everything is going to turn out fine but do not underestimate the importance of your role in helping her through labour. Even the simple things will make a difference. So go on, give her a cuddle as you marvel together at your baby's rapid development over these coming weeks.

FACTS ABOUT YOUR BABY'S DEVELOPMENT

If your baby was born at 28 weeks, he would have a 90 per cent chance of survival – and these odds improve as the weeks go on. Although you may be eager to finally meet your baby face to face, there is still a lot going on inside.

▶ Around week 28, your baby's eyelids will partially open and eyelashes will have formed. He's about 25.5 cm long and weighs approximately 1 kg (2.25 lb).

▶ The bones are fully developed by week 29, though still soft and pliable.

▶ At week 30 the eyes are wide open for a good part of the day, whilst red blood cells have started to form in his bone marrow.

▶ We're only at week 31 but the nervous system has developed enough to control its own body temperature. Wow!

▶ If that isn't impressive enough, at week 32, even though your baby's lungs haven't fully formed, he's practising his breathing.

▶ Around week 33, your baby's pupils can constrict, dilate and detect light.

▶ At week 34, the fingernails have reached the fingertips.

▶ The baby's limbs get chubby from the week 35 mark, and he'll put on about 225 g (0.5 lb) every week for the next month.

▶ By week 36, the baby takes up most of the amniotic sac so it'll be hard for him to give your partner a punch but there should be lots of kicks, stretches and wiggles.

▶ At **week 37** the baby is at early term – his organs are able to function on their own and his head may well descend into the pelvis area ready for the birth.

▶ Get ready to go gooey. Around **week 38**, the baby is developing a firm grasp.

▶ Also helping your baby gear up for life after labour is the placenta, which by **week 39** is supplying your baby with antibodies to help fight infections in the outside world.

▶ This is it. **Week 40** means the due date is here. Your baby will be around 45–50 cm long and weigh about 3 kg (6.5 lb) – so is ready to be born. But healthy babies come in all sizes.

WHAT HAPPENS TO YOUR PARTNER'S BODY?

As the third trimester begins, you will probably think that your partner can't get any bigger – but she will...

▶ As the uterus expands **between 29 and 32 weeks**, your partner's tummy will tighten, leading to more of those Braxton Hicks contractions. Its expansion beneath the diaphragm, the muscle just below the lungs, means she will easily become breathless – in other words, it may be an effort for her to do very much.

▶ From about **33 weeks to 37 weeks**, her breasts will begin to leak colostrum, the precursor to breast milk, and the belly button might pop out. Meanwhile the pelvic ligaments are softening in readiness for the birth.

▶ The good news is that from **37 weeks** until the birth, weight gain will slow down and breathing will get easier as the baby moves closer to the pelvis. The trouble is, it will push down on your partner's bladder so she'll need to go to the toilet more often than ever.

DEALING WITH THIRD TRIMESTER CONDITIONS

It's only just been said but it is worth saying again. From now on until the birth, it is going to be quite an effort for your partner to do anything too physical without quickly getting out of breath, especially in the early part of this trimester, so make sure you help her do things where you can.

Other things to watch out for include:

GESTATIONAL DIABETES

What causes it? Sometimes during pregnancy, women develop higher than normal levels of glucose in the blood and the insulin hormone cannot bring it under control. So this type of diabetes develops and it is only detectable from around 24 weeks. Symptoms include:

▶ A dry mouth with increased thirst

▶ A need to urinate at night

▶ Tiredness

▶ Recurring infections

▶ Blurred vision

Is it treatable? Yes – the condition affects around 18 in 100 pregnant women and once diagnosed is easily monitored and treated through diet and exercise. Your partner will be taught to measure her blood glucose levels and told how often she should do it. Then it is a case of adhering to the following guidelines:

▸ Eat regular, balanced meals – this means food that includes a starchy carbohydrate with a low glycaemic index (GI) such as grainy breads, pasta, rice, new potatoes, sweet potatoes, porridge oats, natural muesli. These will help her absorb the carbs more slowly, keeping glucose levels stable between meals.

▸ Eat more vegetables but don't overdo the fruit – limit the latter to one small serving at a time as it is high in natural sugars.

▸ Limit sugar and sugary foods.

▸ Eat a small amount of unsaturated fats every day – e.g. avocado, a handful of nuts and seeds.

▸ Exercise.

Your partner may also be given medication if the doctor doesn't think diet and exercise will do quite enough. Don't worry – she and the baby will be closely monitored for the rest of the pregnancy.

Will she have diabetes forever? No. Her glucose levels should return to normal after birth – she'll be tested again around six weeks after the birth. There is a slightly increased chance of developing type 2 diabetes at some stage of her life but she will now have a yearly test.

BACK PAIN

This intensifies in the third trimester because the pregnancy hormones relax the joints between the bones and the pelvic area. Here are some things you can do to help:

- ▸ Get your partner to lie on her side or lean forwards over the back of a chair and gently massage her lower back.

- ▸ Have a steady supply of heating pads and ice packs in the house. Warm (but not hot) baths or jets of water from the shower head may also ease discomfort.

- ▸ Always let her have the seats with good back support.

- ▸ Exercising in water is thought to ease back pain in pregnancy and some swimming classes hold aquanatal classes with qualified instructors.

Contact your GP if the pain is particularly bad and persistent or if it is accompanied by other symptoms such as pain and a grinding or clicking sensation around the pubic bone which may mean she has symphysis pubis dysfunction, where the joint at the front of the pelvis becomes less stable.

SPIDER VEINS, VARICOSE VEINS AND HAEMORRHOIDS

Your partner's increased blood circulation might cause tiny red veins on the skin, or spider veins. She might also develop blue or reddish lines beneath the skin – particularly in the legs – which are known as varicose veins. Varicose veins have a tendency to swell up in the rectum, and these are called haemorrhoids or piles.

All of these things can occur in people (male and female) who are not pregnant but pregnancy makes a woman more susceptible to them. Here's what you can do to ease the discomfort:

▶ Get her a foot rest to elevate the legs.

▶ Buy support stockings.

▶ Make sure she's eating lots of fibre and drinking plenty of water to help prevent constipation, which makes haemorrhoids/piles worse.

▶ Don't let her stand for long periods.

Speak to the GP first if the haemorrhoids worsen and they may prescribe a suitable ointment.

SWELLING

The uterus puts a strain on the veins that return blood from the feet and legs and this may cause swollen legs, ankles and feet. Swelling in the legs, arms and hands can place pressure on nerves, causing numbness and tingling – this is nothing to worry about.

Reduce swelling by always getting something to help prop up her legs and make sure she doesn't sit with her legs crossed. Also no standing still for too long.

FREQUENT URINATION

This will be the case late in the third trimester, to the extent that she may leak water when she laughs, coughs or sneezes. She'll find ways to deal with this but it is worth just reiterating that you should look out for signs of a urinary infection which could increase the risk of pre-eclampsia and other complications.

Things to look out for are: passing water even more frequently, pain when passing water, fever, backache.

Other things that recur from earlier trimesters include: Braxton Hicks contractions, heartburn, continued breast growth.

Top Tip

As your partner's bump grows, she will be saying goodbye to seeing her toes easily for a number of weeks. If you can help her trim and paint her toenails, you will be stacking away enough brownie points to last until your baby hits his teens.

ANTENATAL CARE

By now your partner – and hopefully you – will be used to going along to antenatal appointments. In the third trimester they may become more frequent but they will mostly be quite quick, with the midwife or doctor simply wanting to check the following:

▶ No sign of heightened protein levels in the urine

▶ Normal blood pressure

▶ The baby is in a good position by feeling the abdomen

▶ The baby is growing normally by measuring the uterus

▶ The baby's heartbeat is functioning well

There is no need for you to attend these appointments, although there is no harm in planning your day off from work around one and then going for a lunch date or to see a film. Make the most of the free time together while you can!

And if the pregnancy is uncomplicated and your partner is in good health, she may not be seen as often as someone who needs to be more carefully monitored.

ANTENATAL CLASSES

Your partner will have most probably booked these classes many weeks ago in the first trimester. Back then you would have filed it in the box in your brain marked 'Oh, that's ages away – forget about it.' Well now, guess what – it's time to open it up and then process in the cog marked 'What is it I'm supposed to do again?'

Essentially the main thing you need to do is make sure you turn up! You may have heard stories about having to hand round knitted vaginas and talk about your feelings of becoming a dad but, hey, if you're feeling nervous, reluctant or silly about going along, well, you won't be the only dad (or mum) in the room feeling that way.

There's nothing groundbreaking or rocket science-esque about the information the class leader is going to impart but it will quite likely answer a few questions that may have been lurking in the back of your mind and put you more at ease with what is about to happen within the next couple of months.

Some of what is covered will be things that you will already be familiar with, such as healthy eating and exercising during pregnancy. Other areas for discussion might be new subjects that you're about to become all too familiar with, such as breathing exercises and relaxation techniques and positions to adopt during labour, and also matters perhaps already covered in the birth plan such as pain relief and intervention techniques.

There is also an opportunity to learn more about life with a new baby, such as feeding your baby and looking after your own health as new parents.

The point is, you might be dreading the whole experience because you'll have to practise breathing exercises in front of complete strangers but try to embrace it and have fun. You may just meet the people who become your lifelong friends, your first real parenthood-related mates with whom years down the line you'll still relate the time when you looked so silly doing said breathing exercises in front of an audience. And that, ahead of any of the practicalities, is reason enough for you to attend.

FOOD

The lists of foods from the first and second trimester chapters still apply here. Heartburn remains an issue in the third trimester and the trick is for your partner to eat smaller portions at mealtimes and have extra snacks throughout the day to make up for this. Avoid citrus fruits and juices, fried and spicy foods.

Although it's good to stay as healthy as possible, the odd bit of comfort food such as a steak pie or a spaghetti bolognese with cheese on top is going to be just the tonic for your partner as she begins to feel the strain of the third trimester and all its limitations. The mental kick of comfort food far outweighs any calorific downside, BUT keep the portions down and serve with vegetables or salad.

> **Top Tip**
>
> Now's the time to invest in freezable Tupperware and double up whenever you cook something that is suitable for freezing (which is usually going to be comfort food). Label clearly and put the tubs in the freezer to get out for easy dinners during the first few weeks of your baby's life when you'll barely feel like buttering toast, let alone cooking a whole meal.

ALCOHOL

Alcohol is still very much a no-no in the third trimester. Far from it being a time when your unborn baby is pretty much fully formed and safe from harm from consuming alcohol, drinking at this stage can still put her at risk of having a low birthweight, physical abnormalities and cognitive issues.

EXERCISE

In some ways, given the size of the bump at the start of the third trimester, just having to climb the stairs to the bathroom is probably enough exercise for your partner for one day. However, the health benefits of your partner doing what exercise she can during this time of pregnancy still apply as they did in previous trimesters. As well as improving cardiovascular fitness, it helps control weight gain and, just as important, improves her state of mind. Think how grumpy you would be if you were to carry the extra weight and endure all the symptoms and conditions that go with being pregnant. Going for a gentle walk or swim with your partner will do wonders to lift the mood and this is probably the best way to help her exercise. Even just 20 minutes a day can help her alleviate stress and make some sense of the many thoughts, emotions and physical qualms that are going through her mind. If you are exercising together, she may even share them with you, which is all the more beneficial. Other forms of exercise she could try:

- ▶ **Body weight workouts** such as squats and wall push-ups to maintain strength

- ▶ **Bicep and tricep work** using 1–2.5 kg (2–5 lb) dumb-bells, to prepare the arms for having to carry the baby around – something that will benefit you, too!

- ▶ **Pregnancy yoga and Pilates** – there will be classes designed for pregnant women which will make it both comfortable and safe for mum and baby in this last trimester. One study showed that yoga decreased levels of anxiety and depression in pregnant women between 22 and 34 weeks so it is worth your partner going to these classes now even if she hasn't done so before.

▶ **Jogging and light running** – only if she has kept these up prior to the third trimester

▶ **Aqua aerobics** may be an easier way to work the muscles than doing weights and again some classes will be designed for the heavily pregnant woman in mind.

Top Tip

Of course, it is all about your partner knowing her limits and not going beyond what she's used to doing. I knew a woman who was doing 30 lengths of the pool and going jogging before coming into work – on the day that she ended up giving birth! But that is because she was used to doing that level of exercise, and in fact was most probably doing less than what she used to do pre-pregnancy.

SEX

The good news is that in the third trimester, many pregnant women actually report an increased libido but, of course, with the ever-growing bump, you might feel less comfortable with the thought of having sex due to worries about whether it might hurt the baby. Well, rest assured, it won't.

That said, you shouldn't be having sex in the third trimester if:

▶ Your partner bleeds after sex – it's probably nothing serious but you should go and see your GP or midwife before having more intercourse.

► Your partner has been diagnosed with placenta praevia, where the placenta ends up lying partially or wholly at the bottom of the uterus between the baby and the cervix. Vaginal sex could cause more serious issues.

► The waters have broken – at this point the bag of membranes in the amniotic sac which protects and cushions the baby in the uterus has torn and so the baby is no longer protected from infection.

Other than that, sex in the third trimester is not only risk-free and perfectly natural, it is also good for you, improving your and your partner's mood and further strengthening the bond between you, which is good for the baby too.

One last point – some people believe that sex can bring on the birth but there is actually no medical research to suggest this is the case.

TRAVEL

As with the latter half of the second trimester, it is best for your partner to avoid long periods of travel. However, if it is necessary, she should be able to get up and stretch her legs at regular intervals – so make hourly stops if you are travelling by car.

Air travel is usually permitted by doctors up until the 36-week mark but if your partner appears heavily pregnant, the airline may refuse to let her fly. Check with the airline before booking.

Top Tip

Make sure your partner has her mobile charged and on her whenever she goes out in case she suddenly thinks she is going into labour.

THINGS TO BUY

You and your partner will have most probably got the big items that you will need for the new baby ordered and sorted and you may even have started working out how to use them (I can't emphasise enough about that car seat!).

As labour day approaches, here are the smaller essential items that you will want to have ready to use, many you will need for just after the birth itself while you are waiting for the doctor to come round and allow your partner (and baby) to go home.

- ▶ **Mattress for the cot** – it MUST be brand new to reduce the risk of cot death.

- ▶ **Cellular blanket for the Moses basket** – these blankets are warm without being heavy on the newborn.

- ▶ **Nappies** – a couple of packs of newborn nappies will keep you going. Premature varieties are available if necessary but if you are suddenly in need of these at the hospital, they usually will have a supply that you can use.

- ▶ **Cotton wool** – baby wipes are a no-no until your baby is six weeks old as they aren't suitable to be used on newborn skin. So it's cotton wool and water until then.

▶ **Muslin squares** – multitasking bits of cloth created and marketed, quite frankly, by an absolute genius. They protect clothes from baby sick, mop up dribbles and provide a soft surface for baby to rest her head.

▶ **Nappy bags** – supermarket value ones are just as effective as the way more expensive scented varieties. It's going straight in a bin, for goodness' sake!

▶ **Value baby bodysuits/sleepsuits and vests** – it's worth buying a few packs of these as the little one will doubtless go through a few every day. Try to get suits that cover the feet – socks and booties rarely stay on a baby's feet and will soon get mislaid.

▶ **Extra layer clothing** – such as lightweight jumpers or cardigans, hats, jackets and coats; even if it isn't particularly chilly outside, newborns take a few weeks to get accustomed to the outside so these layers are necessary. And so socks and booties – if you can keep them on – are particularly useful for trips outside.

▶ **Dummies** – deciding whether to give your baby a dummy remains a hotly debated topic. Pros include: protection against cot death; it helps the baby pacify himself; and easier weaning – far easier to stop a baby using a dummy than his thumb. Cons include: you're more likely to mistake a need for nutrition-based suckling for the desiring of a dummy; it may cause speech problems in later childhood; and it can make the teeth grow oddly. It's up to you to read up on all the facts and decide.

▶ **Items needed for breastfeeding** – e.g. nursing bras and breast pads. Your partner may want to invest in a breast pump so she can store her milk for you to feed to the baby while she rests.

It can cost between £50 and £100 for a good electric one, though manual ones are a lot cheaper.

▸ **Formula milk** – if, for whatever reason, your partner is unable to breastfeed then you are going to want a backup. And it's a great way to feel involved if you actually do the bottle-feeding.

▸ **Microwaveable bottle steriliser** – quite possibly the best £20 you'll spend is this device that you can use to sterilise four bottles, and other baby stuff that needs sterilising like breast pads and dummies, in under two minutes.

REUSABLE NAPPIES

If you are opting to use reusable nappies, you are going to need at least 15 to use in rotation and plenty of (non-bio) washing detergent. A newborn can get through between ten and 12 nappies a day, sometimes more. You'll also need a bucket and nappy liners.

There are disposable nappies on the market that are kinder to the environment if you are concerned about your carbon footprint.

Top Tip

Do your research before you decide which nappies to opt for, and have a pack of disposable nappies to hand if on the second day of paternity leave you are unloading the second load of washing at midnight and suddenly think, 'Stuff this!' In the first few months of your baby's life, you are going to have enough to do without an extra load of washing every day. That's eating into what little sleep time or cup of tea time you have.

EXTRA THINGS NEEDED FOR A HOME BIRTH

If your partner has opted for a home birth, then you have to prepare for your home being turned into a mini maternity ward for a day or longer. A few weeks before the due date, a midwife will bring round a birth pack containing all the bits and pieces they will need. Additionally, it is advisable that you invest in the following:

▸ Plastic sheeting to protect your floor, bed or sofa

▸ Old towels and sheets to cover the plastic sheeting

▸ A few containers, in case your partner is sick during labour

▸ Warm blanket in case she gets cold

▸ Collect old newspapers and sheets or towels to create a covered path between where she labours and gives birth and the toilet

▸ A desk light so the midwife can examine your partner's vagina for tears and also check all is well with the baby

▸ A portable heater to help keep the newborn warm

▸ Clean towels and baby blankets for the newborn

▸ Bin liners for dirty linen and for rubbish

Nearer the time, make sure you have all this to hand and ready to roll out for the labour.

Top Tip

At baby bath time, nothing beats one of those baby towels with a corner that fits over their head so you can easily and securely wrap them in the rest. They'll use it for years!

PATERNITY LEAVE

A quick reminder that, if you haven't already done so, you'll need to give your employer at least three weeks' notice of when you intend to take your paternity leave, possibly in writing. Of course, you cannot know the due date for sure, but keep your boss and HR department up to date of any developments that might lead to an earlier birth.

HOW TO PREPARE FOR LABOUR DAY

Do you know what? Your partner has already done a lot of the hard work to ensure things go smoothly on the big day – and no doubt you have helped too. There are, however, a few practicalities that you'll need to have sorted for the moment your partner goes into labour:

GET THE RIGHT CONTACT NUMBER

This is the first point of contact for your midwife or the hospital where your partner is booked in to have the baby. It's highly likely your partner would have committed this to memory, so make sure you do too. Put it in your mobile, write it by the phone, whatever it takes.

THE ROUTE

By now your partner – and hopefully you – will be used to the hospital where your baby will make his first appearance but do you know the best way to get there? Is there a shorter route or one more likely to be blocked by traffic at certain times of the day? Do your research and test them out!

PARKING

Where do you park? Do you have to pay? There might be special dispensation which the midwife may mention at the antenatal classes. Ask if not. You may have a certain period of time before you have to pay. Then make sure you have the right change in the car that you do NOT touch until the big day.

THE CAR

Always make sure there is enough petrol in the car to get you to and from hospital.

Check the oil regularly and triple make sure you haven't left the lights on – anything to minimise the chances of breaking down en route to hospital.

No car? Or in case of emergency? Or if you've had a drink? Keep a handful of reliable cab numbers in your mobile – and keep this charged at all times!

THE HOSPITAL BAG

Perhaps the most important thing to do in the run-up to the due date is have a hospital bag fully packed and waiting near the front door for you to pick up on your way out of it. Your partner will probably be sorting this out well in advance according to her preferences but in case you have to sort a bag in an emergency, then don't forget the following for her:

- ▶ The birth plan and maternity notes – keep these notes at the top of the bag as you'll need them first when you arrive at the maternity unit

- ▶ Dressing gown, slippers and socks

- ▶ Nightdress or T-shirts – comfortable to wear in labour

- ▶ Massage lotion or oil in case she wants a massage during labour

- ▶ Lip balm as lips can get dry during labour

- ▶ Anything special the birth plan requires, such as a birthing ball. Inflate in hospital – you may want to pack a pump!

- ▶ Hair clips and/or bands if your partner has long hair

- ▶ Pillows – the hospital may not have enough. A special cushion that she uses is a nice touch.

- ▶ Mobile phone and charger (hers and yours)

- ▶ Digital camera in case the phones don't suffice (and spare SD cards!)

- ▶ Things to keep her (and you) entertained: books, magazines, computer tablets

- ▶ If you're bringing CDs to play during birth, check the ward has CD players – if not, pack your own. These days it's probably better to use MP3 players – less to pack!

▶ Drink and snacks to keep you refreshed – enough for both of you

▶ Hand-held fan or water spray to cool her down during labour

▶ Swimwear if she is going into a birthing pool – feel free to pack your own too!

▶ Bendy straws to help her drink during labour

▶ Comfortable shoes for you – you may be doing a lot of pacing

▶ Change of clothes and going home outfit

▶ Her toiletries bag – make sure she keeps this fully stocked and you don't forget things like toothpaste, toothbrushes, shower gel, shampoo and conditioner to help her feel human again after the birth

▶ Other things to remember for after the birth include: leaflets on breastfeeding given at the antenatal classes and accessories like nursing bras, breast pads, maternity pads (a few packs), eye masks and earplugs to protect her from a noisy, bright ward. Also a change of knickers – old, cheap knickers or even disposable ones.

▶ And for the baby you'll need: two or three sleepsuits and vests, baby blankets, nappies, wipes, muslin squares, socks or booties, a nice going home outfit and a hat and jacket for a colder day. Oh, and make sure that car seat is all ready in the car!

Suffice to say, you may need two bags – maybe a bigger holdall (don't make it too heavy) and a rucksack for the smaller items. Be organised and maybe pack larger items like pillows or birthing balls separately – but don't forget them!

So everything's sorted and it still feels like an eon that you have been waiting for the baby to arrive, right? The due date has come and gone and it's increasingly uncomfortable for your partner for all manner of reasons. My only advice would be to make the most of any extra time that your baby is allowing you to spend together doing simple coupley stuff like enjoying a meal together and watching a whole film uninterrupted (well, apart from a few toilet breaks). Oh, and sleep, although, sadly and somewhat unfairly, this also becomes increasingly uncomfortable for your partner to manage.

Rest assured, parenthood is just around the corner. Go on, don't be scared now, turn the page…

CHAPTER 5
BIRTH AND BEYOND

We've all heard the stories of people who give birth in car parks, taxis or in the dairy aisle of the supermarket, but all being well, your partner should have enough warning to get herself in a sensible place in time for the baby's arrival. It is important for her to have her mobile phone handy when she is out and about, though, so she can get help straight away if she needs it – and to call you!

THE THREE STAGES OF LABOUR

The best way to prepare for what your partner is about to go through is to understand what actually happens as the baby embarks on its first incredible journey. It happens in three stages:

1. **Dilation** – contractions will be making the cervix soften and open up (or dilate). It needs to be approximately 10 cm dilated for the baby to be able to pass through. The process can take some hours before your partner is in what midwives call 'established labour' – and even then that only means the cervix is 3 cm dilated. From there it could take anywhere between six and 12 hours to reach full dilation. It is important for your partner not to push until full dilation to avoid tearing the cervix and other complications.

2. **Pushing** – once the cervix is fully dilated, then your partner is safe to go with the urge to push. The midwife should confirm this and help guide your partner into a comfortable position to deliver the baby.

3. **The placenta** – the baby safely delivered, your partner will still be having contractions until the placenta also comes out. It is likely at this point that the midwife will give your partner an injection of syntocinon into her thigh to speed up the process. The drug makes the womb contract and also helps prevent heavy bleeding.

INDUCING LABOUR

Should there still be no sign of labour starting by week 42, then your midwife will speak to your partner about inducing the birth. The first option here is a membrane (or cervical) sweep, where the midwife or doctor sweeps their finger around the cervix to separate the membranes of the amniotic sac from the cervix. This separation releases hormones called prostaglandins which may kick-start the labour. It will cause some discomfort and possibly bleeding afterwards.

If the sweep doesn't work, then your partner will be offered an induction of labour. She'll be admitted to the hospital maternity unit and have a tablet (or pessary) or gel inserted into the vagina. It could take a while and she may be allowed to go home but you should contact the midwife when the contractions begin – or if she has none after six hours, at which point she may have to go in for another tablet.

Sometimes a hormone drip is given to speed up labour but this can take between 24 and 48 hours to work.

Inducing the birth may be something that the midwife will suggest earlier than the 40-week mark if your partner has a medical problem (such as high blood pressure) or there is a complication with the baby (if she isn't growing as fast as she should be).

It's a fairly common process, with 1 in 5 labours being induced in the UK every year. It is likely the labour will be more painful than a labour that starts on its own, with a higher percentage opting for an epidural – but all pain relief methods are still available.

LABOUR SIGNS

For the other 4 in 5 labours, though, the process will begin naturally, so let's rewind a little. You're all packed and ready, and the due date has come (and probably gone). How is your partner going to know that she is in labour? Well, she'll have more of an idea than you, obviously, but just to keep you up to speed, here are the most likely signs:

- ▶ **Strong, regular contractions** – at some stage when your partner suspects she might be in labour, she will ask you to time them; another reason to keep the mobile charged so you can use the stopwatch facility. If the contractions are strong, regular and painful and lasting for more than 30 seconds each time, then labour may have started.

- ▶ **The 'show'** – during pregnancy, a plug of mucus is present in the cervix and just before labour starts, or in early labour, it comes away and is passed through the vagina, either whole or in several pieces. It will be pink in colour as it will be bloodstained –

if your partner is losing more blood at this point, call the hospital/midwife straight away. Not all women have a show.

- ▶ **Waters breaking** – this is when the baby breaks through that bag of fluid called the amniotic sac in which she has been living for the last few months, causing the fluid to flow out of the vagina. It usually happens during labour but sometimes happens before labour starts. Your partner should have a sanitary towel (not a tampon) to hand if she is going out. The waters may be a little bloodstained but if your partner is losing a lot of blood, or the waters are smelly or coloured, contact your midwife immediately.

- ▶ **Backache** – or an achy feeling similar to one your partner might get during her period.

LABOUR DAY

The first thing to do when you suspect your partner might be in labour is not to panic. Control the rush of emotions that may suddenly form inside you and stay calm and level-headed. Easier said than done, I know, and I was far from calm myself until my wife said precisely the first thing that you should always do: 'Let's call the midwife.'

WHEN SHOULD WE HEAD TO HOSPITAL?

The general advice from the NHS as to when to go to hospital is if the waters have broken or if the contractions are:

- ► regular

- ► strong

- ► lasting about 45–60 seconds

- ► about five minutes apart

Hence why it is important to be doing those timings. Even if labour has started, the midwife might consider it too soon for you to get to the hospital. They don't want to get people in too soon as the labour could be a long one, although if it is your partner's first pregnancy, it is more likely they will get you in sooner to prevent worry. Also if the waters have broken, they'll probably want your partner to come in to be checked, especially if it is her first pregnancy – and from there, it is extremely likely that you'll stay!

The call to the midwife is also a time for them to check all is fine with the waters that may have broken or the show that might have presented itself. From speaking to your partner, they will have a good idea of whether you should make your way to hospital imminently or call back when you have further indication that something is happening.

It's also important to keep them updated because they can start making sure there is a delivery suite available for you when you arrive. So even when you're 100 per cent sure the baby is coming and you're heading out the door, ring them first to let them know you are on your way.

Top Tip

The waters breaking may not be the call to arms that first-time dads may feel it is.

When my wife's waters broke, we were just about to serve up a hotpot for dinner. The midwife said to take our time to enjoy that and then head to hospital later that night.

WHAT TO DO IF THEY SAY TO WAIT TO COME IN

If the waters haven't broken and they ask you to call back, be sure to do the following:

▶ Keep timing any contractions – any significant changes, call the midwife back.

▶ Help your partner with relaxation and breathing exercises that you learnt at the antenatal class. These will help her resist the urge to push which can cause complications as well as tear the cervix.

▶ Massage her back as this is a good way to relieve the pain.

▶ Make sure she keeps her strength and energy up for the labour by continuing to eat and drink (isotonic drinks being good), even if she doesn't feel like it.

▶ Try to get some sleep – a warm bath or shower may help your partner to relax.

▶ Encourage your partner to keep gently active and upright as this will help the baby move down into the pelvis and help the cervix to dilate. Alternatively sitting on a birthing ball may help.

ADMISSION TO THE MATERNITY WARD

You'll know how to get there and where to park, right? And you'll know if and when you need to pay any parking charge – make a good note of any time when you may need to go and get another ticket and don't leave it until the last minute because you won't know what is going to happen. Choose an appropriate time to nip out for 15 minutes but do your best to make it back in ten!! A 24-hour ticket will cover all bases here.

Head to the maternity ward and have those maternity notes ready to hand. This should make the admission process straightforward and quick and the staff will endeavour to get your partner to a delivery room so she can get settled and as comfortable as possible.

Then at the earliest opportunity a midwife will:

- ► Check your partner's pulse, blood pressure, temperature and urine.

- ► Feel the abdomen to check the baby's position and also listen to and record its heartbeat.

- ► Examine your partner to see how far the cervix has opened.

In turn you should:

- ► Show the midwife the birth plan so they can do their best to respond to your partner's wishes.

- ► Ask any questions either of you may have.

The midwife will return at regular intervals throughout the labour to repeat the checks. In fact, the baby's heartbeat will most probably be checked for one minute every 15 minutes and your partner could even be hooked up to a cardiotocography (CTG) machine so it can be monitored electronically. If they cannot get a good trace, they may even use a clip that can be inserted over the baby's head, if the waters have already broken. Don't be afraid to say if your partner doesn't feel comfortable with any of these methods.

In fact, in general, never hold back from anything you want to ask – the midwife will always have time to answer.

WHAT SHOULD YOU DO TO SUPPORT YOUR PARTNER DURING LABOUR AND BIRTH?

The short answer to this question is 'Whatever she asks!' But actually she will have other things on her mind than to always be thinking of what you can do for her at the very moment she might need it. So here's a good list to commit to memory:

► In the early stages, your main task is to keep her company and occupied with different things to read or a new playlist in her MP3.

► Keep her calm, hold her hand and offer reassurance.

► Massage her back and shoulders and help her move into different positions; anything to make her more comfortable – so don't forget those cushions and birthing ball.

▶ Help her utilise other things that you have ensured are on hand to make the birth easier – such as a birthing pool. Go on, get your trunks on!

▶ Suggest she has a warm bath or shower – it's probably against hospital policy for you to get in too but make sure you are in shouting distance!

▶ As labour progresses and the contractions strengthen, remember those relaxation and breathing techniques.

▶ Help the midwife and doctor follow the birth plan as closely as possible, including making sure pain relief requests are met.

▶ Tell her what is happening as the baby is being born.

Do not hesitate to contact the midwifery staff for assistance or if you have any questions. Don't rely on the call button by the bed – go out to the reception desk if no one is coming to your aid. They won't mind, they're just busy.

Top Tip

The best place for you to be, as you'd expect, is at your partner's side, holding her hand no matter how much she squeezes it, offering encouragement and reassurance no matter how much swearing and abuse she may throw back at you. She may turn the air blue but the midwives will have heard it all before, probably earlier on in their shifts!

It doesn't matter if you can't remember much from the antenatal class; no one is expecting you to be an expert. Your main role is to say things like, 'You're doing a great job… keep it up… everything is going to be fine.'

THE BIRTH

In the early stages of labour at the hospital, you may have had moments where you thought the midwives weren't checking on your partner enough. Rest assured, when the midwife examines her and gives the news that her cervix is 10 cm dilated – or close to it – then you'll soon be made to feel that your partner is the centre of attention. If you have chosen to keep abreast of what is going on down there, then it is likely you'll be able to see the baby's head at this point. This is it…

A second midwife will most probably arrive and both midwives will attend to everything that needs doing as the baby makes its final descent. They will also guide your partner as to when exactly she needs to push.

And then, perhaps before you know it, the baby will come out and, very quickly, a midwife will place it on your partner's chest for her to hold. This sounds too fast a summary but it really will seem to happen like that, as though someone has finally thought to end your partner's ordeal by pressing the fast forward button.

Congratulations! You're parents!

EMERGENCY CAESAREAN

If a vaginal delivery poses a significant risk to your partner or your baby, the midwife and doctor will decide with your partner whether an emergency Caesarean might be the safest option. Reasons might include:

▶ The baby isn't getting enough oxygen and a vaginal birth would take too long

▶ The labour is not progressing – in spite of what your partner is doing, the baby may be struggling to move along the birth canal

▶ Your partner is experiencing a lot of vaginal bleeding in labour

▶ The method of inducing is unable to produce enough contractions for a vaginal delivery

In some emergency situations, the baby may need to be delivered within half an hour – and a Caesarean is the safest way to do this.

WHAT HAPPENS NEXT?

Your eyes will pretty much be focused on this amazing little person who has suddenly appeared. They may be smeared in gunk (that's the vernix) and slightly bloody, but that's your baby, that is.

After your partner has had skin-to-skin contact with the baby, the cord will be clamped and cut – see, those two words alone make me not regret having declined to get involved in this process, but if you have elected to do so, go for it!

The baby will be dried to stop them from getting cold and then your partner will be able to have her first proper, lengthy cuddle. She can ask for the baby to be cleaned up and wrapped in a blanket but, hey, she's waited this long. Then it'll be your turn for a cuddle and a gaze and probably one heck of a smile as you hold your baby for the first time.

Incidentally, there will be a protruding, slightly strange-looking umbilical stump on the baby's navel where the placenta was once connected, just to warn you. It'll fall off within a few weeks.

Your baby will love being close to your partner – and you – so soon after the birth, so be sure to enjoy this moment and ignore anything going on around you. If there is reason for you to know anything, the midwife will interrupt you and keep you informed of what is going on at all times.

Equally there may be a delay in getting you both this first cuddle. The baby may need mucus clearing from his nose or mouth, or she may need additional help with breathing – in this case, she will be taken to a corner of the room and given oxygen.

Rest assured, you will be kept informed on what is happening and your baby will be returned to you as soon as possible.

After you have had a little time with your baby, a midwife or paediatrician will examine the baby, then weigh and possibly measure her, before issuing her with a band with your partner's name on.

You will be offered an injection of vitamin K for the baby which is the most effective way of helping to prevent a rare haemorrhagic bleeding disorder. If you don't like the idea of the baby receiving an injection, oral doses are available but further doses will be needed.

Your partner will also be examined for cuts and tears. Small tears are left without stitches because they will heal better but larger tears will need stitching. This will be performed under a local anaesthetic – or a top-up of the epidural – so your partner should still be able to cuddle the baby while the treatment is carried out.

Of course, if your partner has had a Caesarean, then the recovery process will be different and we will cover this in the final chapter.

HOW LONG WILL MY PARTNER AND BABY STAY IN HOSPITAL?

If all is well, it shouldn't be longer than 24 hours when your partner and baby will be able to come home. In fact, it could well take less time than that, depending on the time of day of the birth.

The midwife will want to check that the baby is breastfeeding properly before considering allowing you home – and only then will a doctor come and discharge you, providing they are happy with mother and baby. In the meantime you may be transferred to a postnatal ward.

You will, of course, have plenty to keep yourselves occupied in that time as you dress your baby for the first time, accustomise yourselves to the feeding process – whether that is breastfeeding, bottle-feeding or both – and then the inevitable nappy-changing process. Just get stuck in. It really isn't that hard!

You will also want to announce the news to family and friends, whether by phone, text, email or social media. You may even welcome a few visitors in to see you – keep these visits as brief as you can because your partner will be tired and need what sleep she can get.

Should it seem likely that they will have to stay the first night, then don't be a martyr and stay in hospital as long as you can get away with – go home and get some sleep! That said, be at the hospital as early you can, ready to help pack up and go home.

You've sorted that car seat, right?

> Some hospitals have photographers who come round the maternity ward, offering to take 'baby's first photo' for you. If your partner is enthusiastic about this idea, then it's possibly because the epidural hasn't worn off. We are well into the twenty-first century and you'll already have a fair few pictures on your phones and digital cameras. There is no need to waste money on a school-photo-style set of pictures that are quite unlikely to be any better quality than ones you can take yourself.
>
> That said, if you are sending out a picture of your partner with your new baby to friends, whether via email or particularly on social media, then check that she is happy with that picture first. I am still being reminded, ten years on, that there was a definite showing of the left nipple in the one that I sent out to our friends – oh, and my wife's grandparents.
>
> *Pete, 34, electrician*

HOME BIRTH

Giving birth at home is not really that much of a different process; once you've made sure you have everything in place to turn your home into a maternity ward for the day, you're following similar steps as you would if you were going to the hospital.

So when your partner thinks she may be in labour, call the hospital. A midwife will come out to you to see how she is getting along, watch her having a few contractions and they may even check how much the cervix is dilated, if that is what your partner wants. If there is still some way to go, it is likely that the midwife will leave and come back – but they will arrange for a second midwife to be present for the baby's arrival.

Keep in touch with the midwife about any developments such as increased rate of contractions or anything that concerns you, no matter how trivial you may feel it is.

Your partner may need to be transferred to hospital if:

▶ the labour is taking a long time

▶ the baby is becoming distressed

▶ your partner requires an epidural

This is actually the case for 45 per cent of first-time mums (but only 12 per cent of mums who've had babies before) so don't be alarmed if it happens to you. If it doesn't, the birth should progress just as it would in a hospital.

If the placenta is having trouble coming away or your partner has a very bad tear, then she might need transferring to hospital. If all is well, though, the midwives will leave you alone with your new baby for a while. One will go while the other will stay to check your partner is OK and to weigh the baby. They will also help with the first feed, if you need it.

Once the midwife sees your partner and baby are comfortable and well, they will clean up the mess and leave. From there, you will receive visits from a community midwife every day for a few days, as you would if you'd had the baby in hospital.

And so you have come to the end of your pregnancy journey. I've done well, too, to get this far and not have called it a 'journey' before now.

For you the adventure is only just beginning. There's a beautiful little baby waiting for her next feed or wanting a change or a cuddle. Probably all three but don't worry – in which order is something you will soon fathom for yourself.

CHAPTER 6
LIFE WITH A NEWBORN

No matter how much you prepare for the birth of your child, there will come a point shortly after he is born when you will be hit with the realisation that, heavens above, you're a dad! YOU are actually a dad. Wow! For the first few weeks you will be learning to cope with the dramatic change in your routine that being a parent entails. There are numerous aspects of it that you will strive to master but don't worry; you will do so far sooner than you think. During this time you will receive plenty of (sometimes unwanted!) advice from people on child-rearing – the way they changed nappies, warmed a bottle, stopped their baby crying, etc. Ultimately, though, you will find your own way of doing things and this chapter explains some of the basics, such as changing a nappy and burping your baby, as well as letting you know what to expect in the way of check-ups and your baby's development over the first three months.

FACTS ABOUT YOUR BABY'S DEVELOPMENT: 0–3 MONTHS

There are many milestones for your newborn to reach, just as there were inside the womb, only now you have the pleasure of being able to witness and record them. You can also detect if, in rare circumstances, anything is not quite right. Remember these milestones are only estimates and, in general, babies catch up with one another at their own pace. However, if you are concerned about your baby not having reached some of them, do not hesitate to speak to your GP or health visitor.

By **one month**, your baby:

- ▶ can gaze at your face and is attracted by black and white patterns.

- ▶ will have fully developed hearing and may turn towards familiar sounds such as your voice.

- ▶ when placed on his stomach, will be able to lift his head briefly and turn it to the side, BUT he will still need to have his head supported when being carried.

See your GP if he:

- ▶ doesn't seem to focus his eyes or watch things nearby or react to bright light.

- ▶ doesn't respond to loud sounds.

By **three months**, your baby:

- ▶ has learnt to smile.

- ▶ is a seasoned impersonator – he will love imitating your facial expressions and trying to mimic the sounds you make through his babbling.

▶ will be able to recognise you from across the room and focus on things of interest, especially faces.

▶ can open and close his hands, bring them to his mouth, shake toys and swat at dangling objects.

▶ when placed on his stomach, will lift his head and chest and make push-up type moves in an attempt to roll over – though he won't quite manage this just yet. He will, however, push down with his legs when held upright – but don't let him support himself yet.

See your GP if he:

▶ cannot support his head very well.

▶ cannot grasp objects.

▶ doesn't smile.

▶ ignores new faces or gets upset by unfamiliar people or surroundings.

> ❝ Always support your newborn's head as their neck muscles aren't yet strong enough to support themselves. Whenever I lifted or carried my newborns, I would instinctively cup my hand around the back of their head, even when their head was resting on my shoulder. ❞
>
> *Alvin, 34, solicitor*

CHECK-UPS AND APPOINTMENTS IN YOUR BABY'S FIRST THREE MONTHS

If you are feeling apprehensive about looking after a new baby, you will be pleased to know that there is a lot of support for new parents and much of it is freely available on the NHS.

Very early on, if not before the birth, you will be given a personal child health record (PCHR) which is a handy way to record the progress of your baby's height, weight, vaccinations and other things of note at various check-ups. It usually has a red cover and is known as the 'red book'. Be sure to take it along to all appointments. You can also add information yourselves, such as milestones reached or any illnesses or accidents your baby has had and the medicines they have been prescribed. In some areas of the country, the red book is available online. Visit www.eredbook.org to find out.

In the first few days of your baby's life, you can expect a daily visit from a community midwife. First and foremost this is to ensure that your partner is recovering well from the birth and there are no further health issues for her and also for the baby, but it is also an opportunity for you to ask any questions.

WHAT WILL MY NEWBORN BE CHECKED FOR?

Your baby will usually be given a hearing test shortly after birth while still in hospital so do check if not and it can be carried out within the first few weeks.

Within 72 hours of birth, your baby will be given a thorough physical examination to check all is well with his eyes, heart, hips and, in the case of a boy, testes.

At five to eight days old (ideally five), your baby will be given a heel prick blood test to screen for a number of rare conditions, including sickle cell disease.

Beyond that, the baton is passed to a health visitor who will conduct a series of health reviews throughout your baby's first year to check their height, weight and other aspects of their development. A health visitor is a qualified nurse who has had extra training and part of their role is to help families, especially those with babies and young children, to avoid illness and stay healthy. These appointments can be carried out at your doctor's surgery, baby clinic or even at your home at a time that is convenient to both you and your partner.

Between one and two weeks, your health visitor will conduct a baby review to help you keep your baby as safe and healthy as possible. They will discuss matters like her feeding routine and offer advice, both spoken and in the form of leaflets that you can peruse at your own pace. They will also offer support with breastfeeding if your partner needs it, and also examine her if she has had stitches. It is also an opportunity to check your partner's general well-being and help her deal with issues such as the baby blues (see p.149). The health visitor will leave you their contact details so you can get in touch with them with further questions at any time or arrange a further appointment.

Around six to eight weeks, you will be invited to bring your baby for a physical examination where, in addition to the checks he had at the 72-hour stage, his weight and head circumference will be measured. You will also have an opportunity to discuss vaccinations available for your baby which begin at around two months of age (see below). Your health visitor will be in attendance too to talk to your partner about her emotional well-being.

VACCINATIONS

There are a number of vaccinations that it is advised that your baby is given throughout the first three months, and beyond. You may wish to attend the first few as a couple to lend support to your baby – obviously there is nothing to fear but even so it still isn't nice for anyone to have an injection, let alone a very small baby. These vaccinations are administered to thousands of babies every year but if you have any concerns, then talk them through with your health visitor.

Most health centres around the UK hold regular immunisation and baby clinics but if these are inconvenient, you can arrange for your baby to be vaccinated by your GP.

Here are the vaccinations your baby will be offered in his first three months:

At **two months**:

- ▶ **5-in-1 vaccine** – a single jab (though administered in three stages) to protect against diphtheria, tetanus, whooping cough, polio and *Haemophilus influenzae* type B, or Hib (a bacterial infection that can cause severe pneumonia or meningitis in young children)

- ▶ **Pneumococcal vaccine** (also known as PCV or 'pneumo jab') – administered in three stages, this protects against pneumococcal infections that can lead to pneumonia, septicaemia and meningitis

▶ **Rotavirus vaccine** – an oral vaccine, administered in two stages, to protect against rotavirus, a highly infectious stomach bug that causes an unpleasant bout of diarrhoea and sickness and sometimes extreme dehydration

▶ **Men B vaccine** – a new vaccine to prevent meningitis targets meningococcal group B bacteria, which are responsible for more than 90 per cent of meningococcal infections in young children. This is administered in three stages.

At **three months**:

▶ **Men C vaccine** – this protects against infection by meningococcal group C bacteria which, like its Men B counterpart, can lead to meningitis and septicaemia. Again administered in two stages.

▶ **5-in-1 vaccine** – second dose

▶ **Rotavirus vaccine** – second dose

DEALING WITH YOUR PARTNER'S POST-CHILDBIRTH HEALTH CONDITIONS

Just as it took time for your partner's body to change to accommodate your baby and all his needs, much will be going on now post-birth to get everything functioning back to its pre-pregnancy state. This is a perfectly normal process and there are ways that you can help your partner recover as well as be able to recognise, in rarer cases, symptoms that might suggest she needs further medical attention.

For the first few days after the birth your partner will be tired and need to rest, even though the excitement and pleasure of having a new baby may give her a certain amount of energy. Help out with the baby whenever you can, especially when she's feeling tired. Here are more specific symptoms to look out for:

THE BABY BLUES AND POSTNATAL DEPRESSION

Having a baby is considered a happy time but it isn't a given that your partner – or indeed you – will feel this straight away.

It is common for new mums to feel emotional and tearful during the first two weeks of the baby's arrival – this is known as the baby blues and affects around 85 per cent of new mums. It can also affect dads.

Don't worry; it is perfectly normal and fairly easy to overcome. Speak to your partner about how she is feeling. It might be that she's feeling regretful that the birth didn't go as she'd hoped – for instance, the baby arrived too quickly for a water birth – or it could be that she is wishing she was still pregnant; sounds strange but the pregnancy was a time full of hopes and dreams rather than the reality of having a baby to look after and all the responsibility that comes with it.

Also bear in mind that she is having to deal with a sharp decrease in hormones following the birth and this could be causing problems with her emotions, not to mention the effect that the demands of a new baby is having on her internal body clock.

Two weeks after the birth, these blues should die down but this is the time you need to be on your guard for signs of postnatal depression. This is a much deeper and longer-term type of depression, which affects 10–15 per cent of new mums and can be anything from relatively mild to severe – but all levels require attention. Do not ignore it.

Some symptoms of postnatal depression such as tiredness, irritability or poor appetite are normal when a woman has just had a baby – but they usually don't stop her from living a normal life. What you must look out for is if your partner is feeling increasingly despondent to the point that looking after herself and the baby becomes too much for her to cope with. Other signs include:

▸ Anxiety and panic attacks

▸ Insomnia

▸ Memory loss or an inability to concentrate

▸ Unable to stop crying

▸ Loss of interest in the baby

▸ Feelings of despair

Even if your partner is experiencing just one of these things, make sure she speaks to the health visitor or ideally sees her GP. Reassure her that it is in no way a sign of her being a 'bad mother'. Postnatal depression is an illness – and often easily treated. Also look out for your own well-being – it is not entirely uncommon for dads to suffer from postnatal depression, and not just if you are the main carer for the baby. So check yourself for any of the above symptoms too.

BLEEDING

It is normal for your partner to bleed for two to three weeks after the birth – and sometimes up to six weeks. The bleeding is known as lochia and is her body getting rid of the lining of the womb. It can come out in gushes or flow more evenly like a heavy period.

Make sure she has plenty of maternity pads to hand to help stem the flow, and be aware of these signs of an infection:

▶ The blood smells unpleasant

▶ She develops a fever

▶ The bleeding stays heavy beyond the first week

▶ Her tummy feels tender

Call the midwife or GP for advice on how to handle these symptoms. In rare cases, your partner might suffer a postpartum haemorrhage (PPH) – where a piece of membrane or retained placenta causes a blockage or the uterus doesn't contract properly after birth. It can happen up to 12 weeks after childbirth. Signs of a PPH include:

▶ Her bleeding suddenly becomes heavy and soaks more than one pad an hour

▶ She passes large clots bigger than a 50 pence piece

▶ She feels faint and dizzy

▶ She develops an irregular or racing heartbeat

Call the health visitor immediately if any of these symptoms occur.

SORE BREASTS AND MASTITIS

Why do sore breasts occur? Usually it is the result of the breasts producing excess milk, which is quite common in the first few days after birth. During this time, the hormone oxytocin is released when the baby starts feeding and later on can cause the breasts to leak, even when your partner just thinks about feeding. This is called the let-down reflex. For some women it can cause a pins-and-needles-like sensation, for others it can be more painful, whilst some don't feel it at all.

What is mastitis? This is where the excess milk is forced out of the duct and into the breast tissue, causing the breast to become red and tender. It will also make your partner feel feverish.

What should I do? In the case of mastitis, she should see a doctor as soon as possible for treatment. You can also prepare her a warm, wet washcloth to place over the affected breast 15 minutes before feeding. Another good thing to remind her to do is to get the baby to switch breasts while feeding.

Is it safe to still breastfeed with mastitis? Yes, because any bacteria in the milk will be destroyed by the baby's digestive juices.

SORE NIPPLES

Be mindful of your partner's nipples and all they have to go through during the first few weeks of breastfeeding. With your baby suckling on them, they'll become very sore, tender and, if your baby has a very strong suck, be liable to crack. Again your partner will know to switch breasts if one is getting sore and to vary the nursing position so a different part of her nipple is compressed each time. It is also best to nurse from the less sore nipple first as when the baby is most hungry, that is when he will suck the hardest.

In addition to this advice, here are a few practical ways you can help:

▶ Help your partner feel as relaxed as possible before a feed and make sure she is comfortable (see feeding section on p.155). If she feels tense, she'll produce less milk and so the baby will suckle harder.

▶ After a feed, she shouldn't button up immediately – briefly exposing her nipples to air will help and it's a good chance to check for any signs of infection, e.g. are they particularly shiny and extra-bright pinkish red?

▶ Regular teabags (e.g. English Breakfast) soaked in cool water and applied directly to nipples after a feed may help to soothe them.

▶ Invest in breast shells (not shields) which will protect the nipples from scratchy clothing between feeds.

▶ Speak to your GP or the midwife about creams to apply, such as a medical-grade lanolin. Avoid oily and petroleum-based products like Vaseline.

HAEMORRHOIDS

Haemorrhoids, or piles, aren't uncommon after childbirth and the best thing you can do to help is make sure your partner has a good diet of fresh fruit, vegetables and salad, plus wholegrain cereal and wholemeal bread to make bowel movements easier and less painful.

AFTER A CAESAREAN

It takes longer for a woman to recover from a Caesarean than it does from a natural birth. In hospital she will be offered painkillers and possibly fitted with a catheter (a small tube that goes into the bladder).

She will be discharged from hospital between two and four days after the birth, depending on the help she has at home. Hopefully you will be on hand to ensure:

- ▶ she gets mobile as soon as possible, getting out of bed and walking around, but make sure she rests regularly and doesn't climb up and down stairs too often as her tummy will still be very sore.

- ▶ she carries out postnatal exercises that will be given to her by the midwife or hospital physiotherapist, BUT normal exercise should definitely be avoided until six weeks at least and only then when she feels able to do so without any discomfort.

- ▶ she takes her prescribed painkillers and also looks after her wound by wearing loose clothing and cleansing gently every day.

- ▶ she doesn't drive until after six weeks – other activities to avoid until then are: carrying heavy things, exercise (see above) and sex.

Your partner should contact her GP or the midwife if she has any of the following symptoms:

- ▶ Severe pain

- ▶ Leaking urine

- ▶ Excessive vaginal bleeding

- ▶ Her wound becomes more swollen, red and painful

- ▶ Shortness of breath

- ▶ Swelling or pain in her calf

These symptoms could be a sign of an infection or a blood clot, both of which should be treated as soon as possible. She may be prescribed daily injections to prevent them.

FEEDING YOUR BABY

In an age where superfoods are all the rage, your partner has the best superfood for your baby on tap – breast milk. Even if she breastfeeds for only the first three months of your baby's life, this will reduce the risk of illness in the first year. There are other benefits to breastfeeding too. The main one is that it is a lovely way for your partner to bond with the baby.

Be mindful that breastfeeding can be emotionally and physically demanding – from sore nipples to doing night feeds – and still the baby might cry. Here's how you can make a difference:

- ▶ Your partner is looking after the baby so why not look after your partner – make sure she has a drink and a snack as she may be feeling a little marooned with the baby in her arms, potentially for a good half an hour.

- Ensure your partner is as comfortable as possible – have cushions and pillows on standby and place them where your partner asks.

- If a breastfeeding session is proving tricky for mother or baby, remind your partner just how amazing this thing is that she is doing for your baby and how she might be able to get help from the health visitor for a particular issue. If it is becoming overwhelming for mother and baby, offer to cuddle and soothe the baby first, allowing the mum to have a break before trying again.

- Take the baby once he has finished his meal. You can burp him, change him if necessary and get him to sleep while your partner enjoys a well-deserved rest.

- Offer to give your partner a break from a feed by suggesting she expresses some milk ready for the next one. There are various manual and electric breast pumps on the market and it will be essential if your partner has to go back to work in the first few months of the baby's life and she is still feeding.

On a more practical level, it's worth remembering these further benefits of breastfeeding:

- No messing about having to sterilise bottles or warm the milk – when this becomes a regular part of the daily routine, you'll miss the days of breastfeeding!

- It costs nothing. That means more money for, well, other baby stuff!

▶ The poo of breastfed babies smells less potent than that of formula-fed babies.

> " Breastfeeding may, at times, make you feel left out and wondering how on earth you will ever get to bond with your baby to the same degree. You may even sometimes resent your baby for taking up too much of your partner's time. Don't worry – all these feelings are perfectly natural and most new dads will experience some, if not all of them at some stage. And yet you can have your role to play in the breastfeeding process. In fact your support is vital.
>
> If you are feeling like a bit of a spare part while your partner is breastfeeding, simply sit beside her and give her a cuddle or stroke her hair while you watch your baby suckle. It's a time when you can all bond, not just mother and baby. The chores can wait. "
>
> *James, 38, post office manager*

TOP FOODS FOR BREASTFEEDING

Here are the best foods for your partner to eat so that she can then pass the goodness on to the baby:

▶ **Salmon** – a powerhouse of nutrition, containing a fat called DHA that boosts the baby's nervous system. DHA is already present in breast milk but levels will be higher in women who include it in their own diet.

▶ **Low-fat dairy products** – whether it's yoghurt or cheese, it's a great source of vitamins B and D and also protein for the baby.

▶ **Brown rice** – the temptation may be to cut the carbs after birth but brown rice is a good way to accumulate calories that will produce the best quality milk.

▶ **Eggs** – whether your partner has them scrambled for breakfast or hard-boiled in a lunchtime salad, they provide essential vitamin D that will help your baby's bones grow.

▶ **Leafy greens** – spinach, broccoli, kale or good old-fashioned greens are a lively gathering of nutrients including vitamin C, iron, calcium (useful if your partner isn't too keen on eating too much dairy), as well as containing heart-healthy antioxidants.

▶ **Fruit** – two to three servings of fruit or fruit juice is ideal for keeping up levels of vitamin C; nursing mums need more of this than pregnant mums to keep energy levels high. Oranges are a quick fix for this, as are antioxidant-rich blueberries.

▶ **Wholegrain bread and cereal** – folic acid is still very much essential for your baby's development and they will be taking a lot of your partner's supply through breast milk. Wholegrain products are usually fortified with folic acid and other vitamins and nutrients, as well as being a good source of fibre.

▶ **Pulses** – dark-coloured beans, such as kidney beans, are a particularly good source of iron and non-animal protein; essential if your partner prefers a meat-free diet.

FOODS TO AVOID WHILE BREASTFEEDING

Foods for your partner to avoid while breastfeeding include fish containing high levels of mercury, such as shark, swordfish or marlin, and limit consumption of tuna to no more than two tins a week, much like during pregnancy. Some mums also swear the tastes of certain foods will put off their baby from feeding – these range from strawberries to chocolate, kiwi fruit to cabbage. Then there are foods that mums will suspect are causing the baby to have a bad reaction or allergy. If this is the case, it will be something your partner will have eaten anywhere between two and six hours before a feed. The best thing is for your partner to keep a food diary and also note down when your baby behaves in a certain way, then speak to your health visitor or GP for advice. Dairy products, for instance, can cause a reaction in some babies.

ALCOHOL WHILE BREASTFEEDING

The good news is that alcohol isn't completely off limits for your partner while she is breastfeeding. She can have one unit of alcohol every so often without it affecting the baby. However, she will need to monitor her intake and know for sure what constitutes one unit as the alcohol will pass through to your baby via her breast milk. One unit, for example, is half a standard 175 ml glass of red wine, one third of a pint of normal strength beer or one 25 ml measure of whisky. If she wants a bit more than this, then she should express milk beforehand so you can do the next feed from the bottle.

In general, it is important your partner is drinking eight glasses of liquid every day, whether it is water or juice or milk. Dehydration is the biggest energy drainer – so your partner should still keep caffeinated drinks to a minimum.

FORMULA MILK

You should already have a supply of formula milk to hand that is suitable for newborns but you will also need:

- ▶ Bottles and teats
- ▶ A bottle and teat brush for cleaning
- ▶ Sterilising equipment

It is vital that you clean and sterilise all bottles and teats before use. A microwaveable steriliser is by far the easiest method – most bottles and teats are suitable for use in microwaves but check. Alternatively, you can boil the equipment in a pan for about ten minutes. It will stay sterilised in a covered pan or microwaveable steriliser for about three hours, so try to do a whole batch in one go.

The easiest formula milk to use is ready-made in cartons but it is more economical to buy the tubs of powder that you can then make up with boiled water – but this, of course, will need cooling down first which will take longer so always have cartons in the house for emergencies.

If you're using milk straight from the carton, you will need to warm it up, either by placing the filled bottle in a bowl of boiling water or briefly heating in the microwave – if using a microwave, be sure to shake the milk after heating to ensure even distribution of the heat (microwaves heat from the inside to the outside).

Whichever way you prepare the milk, you will need to test the temperature before giving it to your baby. Your wrist is the best place to do this as the skin there is thinner than on the hand. If it is on the tepid side of being warm (rather than being hot), then it is ready! You will soon develop an instinct for this and learn exactly how long the microwave takes to get the milk to the required temperature but, even so, ALWAYS test it!

Don't worry if it takes some time for your baby to feel comfortable with you bottle-feeding him. It is just as new an experience for him as it is for you and you may need to experiment with different size or shaped teats before you find the one that your baby is happy with. Bear in mind, though, if your baby is crying, it could be that he needs burping…

HOW TO BURP A BABY

Soon after your baby's birth, you may think your baby is smiling at you but it will, in actual fact, be wind. It's not a cliché – babies tend to swallow air while feeding and this can make them feel full and uncomfortable. More so when they are bottle-fed because they have no control over the flow of milk from the bottle, whereas on the breast they can suckle at a slower pace. The discomfort will make him cry and swallow even more air so always have this wind in mind when you are bottle-feeding him so you can relieve him of it at the earliest opportunity.

Have some muslin squares at the ready because he is almost certainly going to bring up some of his feed at some stage, so always be prepared. Here are the best ways to wind your baby:

- ▶ Hold your baby over your shoulder so his bottom is supported with your arm. Then with your other hand, gently pat and rub his back to encourage him to burp.

- ▶ Position your baby face down on your lap with his head over your knee – hold him in place with one hand and gently pat and rub his back with the other.

- ▶ Sit your baby up against your tummy, carefully lean him forward, wrapping your arm around him so his chin rests on your arm, then gently pat and rub with the other.

- ▶ Only wind him at convenient breaks, i.e. when he comes off the teat or is finished feeding – otherwise, if he is whisked away from his meal, he is likely to cry and swallow more air than he otherwise would.

- ▶ Keep trying; even switch positions if one isn't working. Sooner or later you will feel and most probably hear (quite impressively in some cases) the magic burp.

When bottle-feeding, you can reduce the chances of wind if you do the following:

- ▶ Keep the baby as upright as possible, much like he would be kept if suckling on the breast.

- ▶ Make sure there is milk covering the teat, so he isn't sucking air.

- ▶ If the flow of milk is too fast, change the teat to a slower flowing one – but not too slow or else your baby will start crying and gulp in more air.

Gripe water is often given to babies before feeding to reduce wind. It's a mixture of herbs, which warm the baby's tummy and break down air bubbles, and sodium bicarbonate, which helps neutralise acid. There isn't any medical evidence to suggest it works but many parents swear by it, so it is worth a try.

If your baby's wind is persistent and regularly causing him discomfort, speak to your health visitor for further advice.

GETTING YOUR BABY TO SLEEP

You may feel that there are many months of sleepless nights ahead but it needn't be like that at all. For the first two months your baby shouldn't be sleeping through the night – although newborns sleep a lot (up to 18 hours a day), they can't sleep for more than three or four hours at a time, day or night.

Between six and eight weeks they start sleeping for shorter periods during the day but longer at night, though they will still need to wake during the night for a feed.

By two months your baby may be able to sleep through the night but chances are it will take a few months. Before you start having palpitations, at three months he should be able to sleep for ten hours at night – and from only six weeks you can begin to establish routines that will help mum, dad and baby all enjoy a good night's sleep as the norm, far more quickly than you may think; so long as you and your partner adopt the same methods. Here's how:

From six weeks (though you can start before) to three months:

▶ Learn the signs that your baby is sleepy. These include the obvious such as rubbing his eyes and yawning and stretching but also the less obvious, such as losing interest in people and toys around him or burying his face in your chest. Also, if he becomes whiny and cries at the slightest thing, this could be his way of saying: 'For goodness' sake, I need some sleep.' Once you think he is sleepy, try laying him down in his Moses basket – you'll get to learn his daily patterns and rhythms and soon instinctively know when he's ready for a nap.

▶ Teach the difference between day and night. It may sound daft but it's never too early to dress them up in day clothes during the day and sleepsuits for the evening. Also there's no need to turn off the radio or not use the vacuum cleaner as daytime should be noisier than night. Chat to him during daytime feeds too and nudge him awake if he nods off. Then at night-time, dim the lights, shut off any noise, stay quiet during the feeds and don't talk to him too much as you change him into his pyjamas. This contrast will help him learn the difference between day and night.

▶ By eight weeks, you can teach your baby to fall asleep on his own, quite simply by giving him the chance to do so. Don't wait until he falls asleep feeding or in your arms – when he's sleepy but still awake, lay him down in his cot and let him fall asleep on his own. This really is the key to developing good sleep habits, and the earlier the better. You may wish to stay with him while he does so but interact with him as little as possible. If you always end up rocking him to sleep, feeding him or singing him a lullaby, all well and good for the first few weeks but then he will come to expect it every night. In the long run it will be better if your baby is able to fall asleep without any help.

At three months and beyond, continue doing the above and:

▶ Establish set times for naps and bedtime, then stick to them. At three months your baby should be napping three times a day for an hour to 90 minutes. Even if your baby doesn't appear tired at these times, he will be ready for sleep.

▶ Introduce a bedtime routine to help get him ready for sleep – give him a bath, get him in his pyjamas, read a story, kiss him goodnight. It doesn't matter what you do as long as you do it in the same order at the same time every night, including weekends.

▶ Begin to establish a daily routine, e.g. certain times for breakfast, play, lunch, snack, even a trip out – you obviously don't have to stick to them rigidly but the more you can do so, the more likely your baby will fall asleep without a problem. Babies thrive on consistency and it helps make them feel secure if they know what to expect.

▶ Try not to let your baby sleep in, as tempting as this may be – wake him at a set time every morning. This may sound like madness but it will help him develop his daily routine and he can easily recharge his batteries at nap time. If you allow him to lie in, you are only making things difficult for nap time.

> Invest in blackout blinds for the baby's bedroom. Then at nap time simply put the baby down in her cot and walk away – and do this regularly. It took quite a time before we realised our baby daughter just wanted to go to sleep and not be comforted. Of course, go back if they keep crying.
>
> *Carl, 42, editor*

HOW TO TELL WHEN YOUR BABY IS ILL

Your baby is obviously too little to tell you when he is ill but fortunately your partner is likely to come preloaded with something called maternal instinct that will quickly detect any signs.

Babies are still developing their immune system so in their first year, they will pick up infections and colds, and most are nothing to worry about. The best thing is to be prepared by doing the following:

▶ Invest in a baby thermometer and learn how to use it.

▶ Stock up on medicines suitable for your baby.

▶ Keep a note of your GP's 24-hour line by the telephone and stored on your mobile.

▶ Keep a first aid kit with baby-friendly creams and plasters so you can quickly tend to any scrapes as he gets older and more mobile.

► Book yourself in for a baby first aid class so you know exactly what to do in more serious cases such as poisoning and choking. Keep any leaflets you are given to hand as a reminder.

HOW TO CHANGE YOUR BABY'S NAPPY

It will be useful to have a practice at doing this before the baby arrives, if only to get an idea of the mechanics behind the brand of nappies you intend to use. Most disposable nappies have adhesive flaps at either side which fasten in the centre, but simply getting to know your way around which part of the nappy fits where – as silly as it might sound – is going to help you when you come to change your first nappy.

The following method will help you cope with each nappy change as smoothly as possible:

1. What you need: changing mat, a few clean nappies, baby wipes (or cotton wool and water for newborns), a nappy bag and nappy cream. You may also need a clean set of clothes for your baby.

2. Prepare, prepare, prepare. Have everything ready to use: the nappy bag already open and close to hand, the nappy laid out ready to slip underneath the cleaned bottom, wipes or cotton wool and nappy cream to the side.

3. If it's just a wee – hallelujah! – but do check to make sure the baby's clothes are still clean and dry. Whisk the wet nappy into a nappy bag, then wipe your baby's nappy area gently – front to back, especially important for a girl – making sure all the nooks and creases are wiped clean.

4. Place a new nappy under the bottom (as quickly as possible, in case of a further wee).

5. If he has a particularly wet nappy, apply nappy cream to outside areas – try not to use too much.

6. Fasten new nappy.

7. Refasten or change baby's clothes.

8. Ensure your baby is in a safe place (i.e. not on the edge of the bed if he is able to roll over) then wipe clean the changing mat and put everything away, disposing of the full nappy bag, then wash your hands!

9. Pick up your baby for a cuddle.

10. If it's a poo, wipe the worst of the damage away and place the dirty nappy in the nappy bag, then wipe the nappy area gently but thoroughly to ensure no poo remains in the nooks and creases.

11. Follow steps 4–9.

> If you're dealing with a baby boy, rest something on his little fella such as a dry baby wipe to stop yourself from getting squirted. Funnily enough, this was one of the things that made me apprehensive about having a boy, and yet it is easy to stop from happening.
>
> *Steve, 41, accountant*

HOW TO WASH YOUR BABY

For the first few days it will be enough to give your baby a quick wash – known as top and tailing – using cotton wool and warm water. Topping means washing his face, neck and hands. Tailing refers to the nether regions, but in the first few days you should also pay particular attention to his umbilical stump which can take anything between five and 15 days to fall away naturally. The umbilical stump will shrivel up and change from yellowish-green to brown or black, when it should drop off naturally. Don't tug at it. Keep it clean and dry to prevent infection and also make sure it isn't covered by the nappy and that your baby wears something loose over the stump.

Here's how to top and tail/wash your baby:

▶ Make sure the room is warm and you have a clean nappy and clothes to hand – and that the towel is ideally keeping warm on a radiator.

▶ Fill a bowl or sink with warm water.

▶ Undress your baby and place him on a clean towel ready for a quick dry.

▶ Dip the cotton wool in warm water and, making sure it isn't too wet, dab your baby's face around the nose and outwards, then dry. Use a fresh piece of cotton wool for each eye.

▶ Repeat with his neck and hands.

▶ Dry each part thoroughly, being sure to include the folds and creases.

▶ Talk to him while you are washing him to keep him relaxed.

▶ Make sure you keep him warm and after the last wash, pick him up and give him a nice warm cuddle in that pre-warmed towel.

MORE THINGS YOU'LL NEED FOR YOUR BABY

Just when you think you have everything you need for the baby, he only goes and starts growing out of a lot of it. Typical! Hopefully you will be given hand-me-downs to take care of a lot of the clothes he'll need as he grows. Toys and books that other parents no longer need for their children should also be welcomed.

Here are a few bigger items that will come in handy for the first few months:

▶ Activity mat (aka baby gyms) – these are soft mats that the baby can lie down on, with a soft bar arching above containing a variety of soft toys for them to look at and later touch and squeeze. It helps facilitate his development and stimulate his senses, as well as providing him with some variety throughout the day. They are also portable and easily folded and tidied away.

▶ Travel cot – once your baby outgrows the Moses basket, this is a worthwhile investment if you are going on your travels and staying overnight with someone who doesn't have anywhere for him to sleep – it also doubles up as a playpen.

> Embrace the charity shops for cheap toys and books – there seems little point in spending a fortune on one toy that they may not play with more than once or twice. This especially applies for your baby's first Christmas – it's fun to buy a few cheap items that you can wrap up for your baby (and then open for her) to add to the festive atmosphere. Charity shop staff usually clean up merchandise but if you are concerned, simply wipe down toys with a warm damp cloth and some baby-friendly disinfectant.
>
> *Gary, 47, actor*

PLAYING WITH YOUR BABY

It is really never too early to start playing games with your baby – in fact it is often the best way to pass the days that you'll be spending with him. Early on, 'play' can be built into the daily routine to help your baby acclimatise to his own body clock – maybe a session in the morning before a trip out in the afternoon.

So what games? There are singing games, of course. These may involve pointing to parts of your baby or doing actions of some kind that will sooner or later raise a smile from him. Here are some simple songs that you will no doubt recall from your own childhood:

▶ **'This Little Piggy'** – a great one for tickles and toe or finger wiggling

▶ **'Itsy Bitsy Spider'** – a great one for actions

- ▶ **'Pat-a-Cake, Pat-a-Cake'** – a classic

- ▶ **'Old MacDonald Had a Farm'** – a great opportunity to make the baby laugh with different noises

- ▶ **'If You're Happy and You Know It'** – clap your hands, pat your knees, whatever tickles your fancy

- ▶ **'The Wheels on the Bus'** – the folk on the bus chatter, the driver says tickets please, the baby wah-wah-wahs... you can improvise!

- ▶ **'Heads, Shoulders, Knees and Toes'** – another classic!

- ▶ **'Pop Goes the Weasel'** – anything with a surprise 'pop' in it is going to be a surefire hit

- ▶ **'I'm a Little Teapot'** – actions for more advanced performers

- ▶ **'The Grand Old Duke of York'** – you can move your baby (gently) up and down to this one

It is also never too early to introduce books to your baby. These could be soft play books that have different textures to feel – again it's never too soon to help your baby participate in feeling these because it will help them to eventually do it themselves. Flappy books are good for the surprises too and often feature simple words for you to repeat to your baby. And if you have an old favourite storybook from when you were a child (mine was *Dogger* by Shirley Hughes), your baby will just love hearing your voice as you read the story aloud. This certainly isn't an activity exclusive to bedtime. It may also inspire you to take your baby along to your local library where they will most probably hold regular storytelling sessions for babies and toddlers.

> *I started singing my son 'The Alphabet Song' from a very early age and playing counting games too. It sounds silly as you think they are too young to take anything in. But the repetition seemed to set my son up for taking more of an interest in learning as he grew into a toddler. Of course, you can never measure just how much of a difference it is going to make in the long term but the point is to never set limits or restrictions on what you can potentially teach your baby.*
>
> *Dan, 37, gardener*

TRAVELLING WITH YOUR BABY

Now you have a baby in tow, travelling is going to be that little bit slower and requires much more forward planning. Gone are the days when you can run for a train or plane at the last minute – although on the plus side many airlines in particular will grant you priority access as a matter of course. On trains it may be more down to you to book a seat or arrive early so you can get a spot with the space that the baby (plus buggy) will require.

However, all that is probably a little further down the line. In terms of your firstborn, it is all going to begin with the…

FIRST TRIP OUT

It is likely you will keep yourselves locked away at home with the new baby for the first few days – especially with your firstborn –

but then you will want to take the big step of going outside with your baby.

It's a trip best taken together with your partner. You don't need to go very far – just round the block via the corner shop is enough of a first adventure – but it's a good opportunity to kick off the going-out routine in terms of being able to put the pushchair up and down, taking time to secure your baby in it properly, and also packing the changing bag with everything you might need on a trip out (even a relatively short one).

Here's what you should always remember to pack in a changing bag:

▸ Spare nappies, along with nappy cream, nappy bags, wipes, cotton wool – and don't forget a travel changing mat

▸ Spare set of clothes, including layers such as cardigans, extra T-shirts

▸ Muslin squares

▸ Sterilised bottles and cartons of formula milk – or anything required for breastfeeding such as nipple shields (again, sterilised) and breast pads

▸ Hand sanitizer in case you've had to do a nappy change in a changing room without a sink

▸ Sun hat and baby sun cream for hot days

▸ Sterilised dummies (if using)

▸ Lightweight blanket for warmth or shade

- Small first aid kit for any scrapes – child-friendly antiseptic cream and plasters should do it

And don't forget to make room for anything you might need – such as wallet, mobile phone and keys – the fewer bags you are carrying will make a trip out with baby much easier.

The more you go out with your baby, the more confident you will become and having everything you need will be second nature. Before you know it you will be heading out somewhere almost every day and it will become part of your baby's routine. It's good for both baby and carer to get out of the house – both get a change of scene and a chance to meet new people and make new friends. Check out the health centre noticeboard or ask your health visitor for information on local baby and toddler groups and also classes aimed at babies such as music, yoga and swimming. Don't forget the library too.

Trips by car will soon be a necessity and by now you will be adept at fixing and unfixing that car seat. It will need to remain rear-facing until your baby weighs 9 kg and then you will be able to make it forward-facing, although as long as your baby can still stretch his legs, it can remain rear-facing for a time.

And why stop at travelling by car? Until your child is two years old, he can travel for free on a plane. Just make sure you pre-book the baby car seat if you're hiring a car at the other end. Check with your GP about any immunisations your baby may need before the trip, as you would for yourselves.

>   " The first few weeks of being a parent can be claustrophobic, especially for the person who is staying at home with the baby all the time. If you're the one going back to work, make sure you give your partner the chance to get out of the house on her own for a bit, ideally every day, even if it is a ten-minute walk to the shop and back.
>
>   Also, if you are heading off on a trip out together, why not give your partner a bit of a break to go round the shops while you take the baby for a stroll. You might like the attention you get. I'll never forget carrying my son around the supermarket in my arms when he was just a few days old, only for all manner of staff and customers to come up and say 'Isn't he lovely!' and have a bit of a coo. It's a good opportunity for father and baby to bond at a time when breastfeeding might be making you feel a little left out. "
>
>   *Alan, 41, writer*

YOUR RELATIONSHIP WITH YOUR PARTNER

There are two ways to look at how a baby might affect a couple's relationship. The usual line is to say that it will leave you with no time for one another and when you do have time together, you'll be completely exhausted.

Although, of course, there is some truth in this, it is better to focus on the other way of looking at it. Having a baby also has you working as a team for a very common, very beautiful good. Sure, you are going to argue and get tetchy with one another, but just be mindful of the circumstances and take time to calm down, talk and resolve the issue.

And when you do end the day exhausted and fall asleep on the sofa together, well, isn't that a pretty nice picture of a good relationship?

As you both get into the routine of being parents, slowly you will find more time for one another – and you will wisely target relatives and friends to volunteer for babysitting duty while you take time out to enjoy a date night. Even if someone can only mind the baby for a couple of hours on a Saturday afternoon, bite their hands off! Any time you get to spend together alone as a couple will help to keep your relationship strong.

Then there is the question of sex. For the first few weeks your partner will be recovering from the birth and you will both be too tired to think about being intimate anyway. As time goes on, though, it may well happen naturally again or you might want to communicate your worries about it. Around 50 per cent of couples wait at least six weeks until they try, with most having tried by about three months, especially if the mother has had a tear or episiotomy. Your partner will want to be careful the first few times to make sure penetration doesn't hurt, so take things steady and listen to her. Before you know it, you'll both be enjoying a healthy sex life – as much as having a new baby permits, that is.

> If, during sex, there are issues making penetration difficult for your partner, she should see her GP as soon as possible. It could be that there is vaginal tearing that happened during the birth that was, for some reason, undetected. Most of the time this isn't the case – such tears are quickly recognised and effectively managed. In the case of my partner, postnatal stitches had healed badly and she needed a small procedure to fix the problem. Don't, for a moment, consider any issues regarding sex unimportant – especially, of course, if you are planning to have another baby.
>
> *Tom, 42, engineer*

The key isn't just about spending time together alone and maintaining a good sex life, it's more about the quality time you spend as a new family. Get to grips with the routine and you will negotiate trips out with increasing ease and on those trips you will create many happy memories that you will think and talk about for years to come.

CONCLUSION

Talk of another baby is a good place to end this book. If you're reading this part before or very shortly after your first baby has arrived, the thought of another may just be too much to bear for the moment.

We started this book discussing the element of fear that every dad-to-be feels upon learning that the baby is on the way. Well, look how far you have come since then. Another baby? Bring it on!

Never mind that you don't know what challenges having two children will mean or the implications it will have on your life. Think of what you once didn't know about being a dad that has now become second nature to you. You learnt it and got to grips with it because you had to – and now you are reaping the rewards every time you hold that cuddly little baby in your arms and he looks up at you and smiles.

And if, for whatever reason, another baby isn't on the cards, facing the unknown is a lesson that you can apply to other aspects of your life, whether it be starting a new business venture or moving to a new area.

In other words, a little fear is good, especially now that the whole pregnancy and parenthood experience has taught you how to embrace it.

DIRECTORY

The following is a list of contact details that you might find useful throughout your partner's pregnancy and beyond. It isn't by any means intended to be fully comprehensive and there will be numerous organisations working on a local or regional level that you might be able to contact for help.

ALCOHOL PROBLEMS

Drinkline
0300 123 1110
9 a.m.–8 p.m. weekdays, 11 a.m.–4 p.m. weekends
Offering support if you are worried about your own or someone else's drinking.

NOFAS (National Organisation for Foetal Alcohol Syndrome)
020 8458 5951
www.nofas-uk.org
Supports people affected by foetal alcohol spectrum disorders (FASD) and their families and communities and promotes public awareness about the risks of alcohol consumption during pregnancy.

FAS Aware

fasaware.co.uk

Provides information, advice and guidance to make informed choices about the effects of alcohol during pregnancy and the detrimental impact on the adults and children throughout their lives.

Addaction

www.addaction.org.uk

UK-wide specialist treatment charity that helps individuals, families and communities to manage the effects of drug and alcohol misuse.

BREASTFEEDING

National Breastfeeding Helpline

0300 100 0212

9.30 a.m.–9.30 p.m. every day of the year

www.nationalbreastfeedinghelpline.org.uk

Web chat service also available on the website.

Association of Breastfeeding Mothers

0300 330 5453

abm.me.uk

La Leche League

0845 120 2918

www.laleche.org.uk

For friendly mother-to-mother breastfeeding support from pregnancy through to weaning.

NCT Breastfeeding Helpline

0300 330 0771

8 a.m.–10 p.m., seven days a week

Baby Café

www.thebabycafe.org

Website which lists its breastfeeding drop-in centres around the UK, mainly in cities.

DISABLED PARENTS

Disabled Parents Network

disabledparentsnetwork.org.uk

A national organisation offering information and support for disabled people who are parents or who hope to become parents, and their families, friends and supporters. For general queries, visit the contact page: disabledparentsnetwork.org.uk/contact/

ECTOPIC PREGNANCY

Ectopic Pregnancy Foundation

0845 070 4636

www.ectopicpregnancy.co.uk

Forum available on the website.

Ectopic Pregnancy Trust

020 7733 2653

www.ectopic.org.uk

GENERAL SUPPORT

National Childbirth Trust (NCT)

0300 330 0700

www.nct.org.uk

Information and support in pregnancy, childbirth and early parenthood. Callers are put in touch with counsellors and/or local and regional contacts for support groups including groups for Caesareans and miscarriage.

Family Lives

0808 800 2222

www.familylives.org.uk

Offers 24-hour support to anyone parenting or helping to raise children, from newborn babies to young adults.

Tommy's – pregnancy support

0800 0147 800

9 a.m.–5 p.m. to speak to a midwife about non-urgent matters

Or email info@tommys.org

HEALTHY EATING

Change4Life

0300 123 4567

9 a.m.–8 p.m. every day

www.nhs.uk/change4life

Advice on ways to eat more healthily during pregnancy and beyond.

INFERTILITY

Infertility Network UK

0121 323 5025

www.infertilitynetworkuk.com

Advice, support and understanding for anyone affected by infertility, information on support groups, and fact sheets.

MISCARRIAGE/STILLBIRTH

Miscarriage Association

01924 200 799

www.miscarriageassociation.org.uk

Information and support for people affected by the loss of a baby in pregnancy.

CareConfidential

0300 4000 999

Offers miscarriage and other baby loss support. Also unplanned pregnancy support.

British Infertility Counselling Association

bica.net

BICA is the only professional counselling association for infertility counsellors and counselling in the UK, seeking to promote the highest standards of counselling for those considering or undergoing fertility investigations and treatment.

Tommy's – bereavement counselling
0800 0147 800

9 a.m.–5 p.m.

Call the helpline to arrange to speak to a trained bereavement counsellor. Or email info@tommys.org

Sands
020 7436 5881

www.uk-sands.org

Supports anyone affected by the death of a baby that has died before, during, or shortly after birth.

The Compassionate Friends
0345 123 2304

10 a.m.–4 p.m. and 7 p.m.–10 p.m. every day

www.tcf.org.uk

An organisation of bereaved parents, siblings and grandparents offering support and mutual understanding to others after the loss of a child, of any age, from any cause. It has a national helpline, with calls answered only by bereaved parents, as well as a comprehensive website.

Child Bereavement UK
0800 02 888 40

www.childbereavementuk.org

Supports families and educates professionals when a baby or child of any age dies or is dying, or when a child is facing bereavement. Alternatively email enquiries@childbereavementuk.org

MULTIPLE BIRTHS

TAMBA (Twins and Multiple Birth Association)

0800 138 0509

www.tamba.org.uk

TAMBA is a charity that directly helps parents of twins, triplets and more to meet the unique challenges that multiple birth families face.

The Multiple Births Foundation

0208 383 3519

www.multiplebirths.org.uk

Advice, information and support to multiple birth families.

PRE-ECLAMPSIA

Action on Pre-Eclampsia

0208 427 4217

9 a.m.–5 p.m. weekdays

action-on-pre-eclampsia.org.uk

Support for pregnant women who have experienced pre-eclampsia and for concerned relatives. Alternatively, email info@apec.org.uk – all emails answered personally and in confidence.

PREMATURE BABIES

Bliss

0500 618 140

www.bliss.org.uk

Confidential advice, information and support to families of premature and sick babies.

POSTNATAL DEPRESSION

House of Light
0800 043 2031
www.pndsupport.co.uk
Support for women and their families suffering from postnatal depression.

Pandas Foundation
0843 289 8401
www.pandasfoundation.org.uk
A support group network for families of women (and men) who are suffering from pre- or postnatal depression.

SMOKING

NHS Smoking Helpline
0300 123 1044
9 a.m.–8 p.m. weekdays, 11 a.m.–4 p.m. weekends
www.nhs.uk/smokefree

QUIT
0800 00 22 00
9 a.m.–8 p.m. weekdays, 10 a.m.–6 p.m. weekends
www.quit.org.uk

TRAUMATIC BIRTH

The Birth Trauma Association
www.birthtraumaassociation.org.uk
Support to all women who have had a traumatic birth experience.

YOUNG PERSON'S SUPPORT

Brook
www.brook.org.uk
Information and support for young people under 25 on sexual health, contraception, pregnancy and abortion.

INDEX

ABOUT THE AUTHOR

Adam Carpenter has worked as an editor and freelance writer on several leading national magazines. Among other titles, he has written for *Practical Parenting*, *Mother & Baby*, *Brides* and *Cornwall Today*. He writes a regular column for *Writers' Forum* and has been a blogger on www.workingmums.co.uk. He also presents a weekly show on CHBN Radio. He lives in west Cornwall with his wife and two children.

adamcarpenterjournalist.wordpress.com

NOTES

NOTES

NOTES

NOTES

NOTES

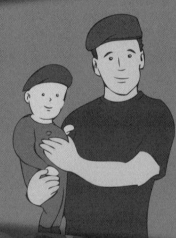

COMMANDO DAD

BASIC TRAINING

HOW TO BE AN ELITE DAD OR CARER

NEIL SINCLAIR

THE BASICS

- Survive the first 24 hours
- Prepare and plan to prevent poor parental performance
- Maintain morale
- Feed, clothe, transport and entertain your troops

FROM BIRTH TO 3 YEARS

Foreword by Dr Jan Mager-Jones MB ChB

COMMANDO
DAD

Commando Dad
How to be an Elite Dad or Carer

Neil Sinclair

£10.99
Paperback
ISBN: 978 1 84953 261 7

As used by Prince William, here's the basic training manual for new recruits to fatherhood!

Attention! In your hand is an indispensable training manual for new recruits to fatherhood. Written by ex-Commando and dad of three, Neil Sinclair, this manual will teach you, in no-nonsense terms, how to:

- Survive the first 24 hours
- Prepare and plan to prevent poor parental performance
- Maintain morale
- Feed, clothe, transport and entertain your troops

And much, much more. Let Training Commence.

THE NEW PARENTS' SURVIVAL GUIDE

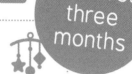

The first three months

Wendy Green

The New Parents' Survival Guide

Wendy Green

£7.99
Paperback
ISBN: 978 1 84953 715 5

Everything you need to know to guide you through your baby's first three months and beyond!

No matter how much you long for and plan for a baby, no one is quite prepared for the impact their new arrival has on their life. This book recognises that no one has a textbook-perfect baby and lets you in on what you can REALLY expect in the first three months. *The New Parents' Survival Guide* is packed with practical advice and simple tips on how to deal with common problems you are likely to encounter, including how to:

- Care for your newborn
- Solve the breast versus bottle dilemma
- Overcome breastfeeding woes
- Calm your crying baby
- Solve sleep issues
- Manage minor ailments
- Take good care of yourself

Have you enjoyed this book?

If so, why not write a review on your favourite website?

If you're interested in finding out more about our books, find us on Facebook at Summersdale Publishers and follow us on Twitter at @Summersdale.

Thanks very much for buying this Summersdale book.

www.summersdale.com